Hypoglycemia For Dummies®

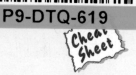

Cheat Sheet

Starting to Recover

When beginning your hypoglycemia recovery program, the most crucial steps can be tough:

- Eat breakfast every day, within 1 to 2 hours of getting up.
- Eat some protein at every meal and snack.
- Eat frequent, small meals and snacks (3 meals, plus 3 or more snacks, or 3 small meals).
- Eat mainly complex carbohydrates.
- Keep sugar and refined flour products to a minimum.
- Avoid caffeinated drinks.

Give yourself time to become accustomed to these changes. Don't rush.

Foods to Choose

You can eat a variety of foods:

- Organic meats, vegetables, and fruits whenever possible
- High-quality protein (fish, poultry, lean meat)
- Fresh fruits, preferably with a meal
- Fresh vegetables, lightly cooked or raw
- Nuts and seeds
- Alternative sweeteners, such as stevia
- Filtered water

Moving Toward a Hypoglycemia-Friendly Lifestyle

These tips can get you started toward the right lifestyle:

- Chew your food thoroughly.
- Stop eating before you feel completely full.
- Sit and enjoy your meals in a relaxed atmosphere.
- Keep your daily food journal (see Chapter 6).
- Take the right vitamins and minerals (see Chapter 7).
- Get plenty of exercise (see Chapter 8).
- Release and resolve stresses (see Chapters 9 and 10).
- Maintain a positive, upbeat attitude (see Chapter 10).
- Ask for help when you need it (see Chapter 12).

Run, Don't Walk, Away from These

Just say no to

- Processed foods
- Fried foods
- Hot dogs, sausages, and deli meats
- Arguments, debates, and unpleasant topics when eating

For Dummies: Bestselling Book Series for Beginners

Hypoglycemia For Dummies®

Cheat Sheet

BESTSELLING BOOK SERIES

Tackling Temptation

Hypoglycemia seems to be about all the things you can't have. Here's some information that can help you beat temptation:

- **Toss it.** Toss out anything and everything that's on the list of foods to avoid. If you need your favorite fix, you'll have to get into your car and drive to the store, or do something equally inconvenient.

- **Breathe.** When you get strong urges to eat something non-hypoglycemically-correct, take in very deep belly breaths. Continue taking in deep belly breaths until the craving dissipates. Aim for at least five minutes.

- **Bathe.** Go take a bath or shower. Water can help clear stagnant energy, and soaking in a hot bath can help relax you.

- **Drink.** Sometimes we have a yen for a certain food when actually we're thirsty. Instead of giving in to your cravings immediately, slowly sip a glass of water.

- **Meditate.** Ask yourself what feeling you're trying to experience by eating the food you're craving. Meditate and bring the feeling into you. Visualize a balloon hovering above your head, and let it expand. Fill it up with all the sensations you want, such as peace, bliss, or healing. The balloon is starting to glow like the sun. Now let the balloon pop, and let its contents cascade down onto you, filling up all the cells of your body. Let your body absorb everything fully and completely.

- **Pause before caving in.** Don't give in to the urge right away. Bargain with yourself. Tell yourself, "I will eat in ten minutes or a half hour".

- **Switch and unbait.** Switch to something that's similar, but without the harmful effects. For instance,
  - Make your own ice cream using cream, protein powder, and an alternative sweetener, such as stevia or sucralose.
  - Make your own chocolate with carob powder and alternative sweeteners.

- **Use alternative sweeteners.** These sweeteners won't trigger a rapid insulin response:
  - Stevia, a natural sweetener made from a South American herb
  - Fructooligosaccharides (FOS) — you win a prize if you can say this word five times quickly
  - Crystallized raw cane juice, a whole food that contains chromium and other nutrient complexes

- **Avoid artificial sweeteners.** Kick aspartame out the window.

- **Get active.** Instead of sinking your fangs into food, do something else.

For Dummies: Bestselling Book Series for Beginners

Hypoglycemia FOR DUMMIES®

by Cheryl Chow and James Chow, M.D.

WILEY

Wiley Publishing, Inc.

Hypoglycemia For Dummies®

Published by
Wiley Publishing, Inc.
909 Third Avenue
New York, NY 10022
www.wiley.com

For general information on our other products and services or to obtain technical support, please contact our Customer Care Department within the U.S. at 800-762-2974, outside the U.S. at 317-572-3993, or fax 317-572-4002.

Wiley also publishes its books in a variety of electronic formats. Some content that appears in print may not be available in electronic books.

Library of Congress Control Number: 2002114829

ISBN: 0-7645-5490-5

Manufactured in the United States of America

10 9 8 7 6 5 4 3 2

1B/RU/QS/QT/IN

About the Authors

Cheryl Chow has been a freelance writer, editor, and journalist for over 20 years, concentrating on health and social issues. She has a diverse writing background, having written for magazines, newspapers, and webzines. She's also done a stint as a broadcast reporter with a weekly spot reporting on the news show "Out and Around" for NHK Radio Japan. She has also translated for the TBS bilingual (Japanese/English) TV news. Chow's works have appeared in such anthologies as *Naming the Daytime Moon, The Broken Bridge,* and *Tokyo Confidential.* She has also written a 30-year corporate history of Dupont-Toray and ghost written a book on Feng Shui.

Chow contributes weekly columns to the *Mainichi Daily News* and has been the editor of *Ikebana International Magazine,* the editor of the Research and Development Department of Time-Life Japan, and the Nippon Foundation. She is a translator of health and business topics and worked as a translation checker for major publications including *Newsweek Japan, National Geographic,* and the *Washington Post.*

Coming from a family with a long line of medical doctors, Chow has always been fascinated by medicine and science. After obtaining a B.A. in psychology from Reed College, she pursued her own studies into the effects of mind over body and vice versa. She has conquered her own bouts with hypoglycemia, fatigue, and other health issues through attention to lifestyle and diet. She has studied t'ai chi, chi kung, ba gua, and meditation from some world-renowned teachers, and has also taught t'ai chi exercises for health.

James H. Chow, M.D., is the medical director of Nippon Clinic. He specializes in emergency and family medicine. Before he went into private practice 16 years ago, he was the director of the emergency department at Mt. Sinai Hospital in Chicago for seven years. As an emergency doctor at one of the busiest hospitals, he has encountered and treated almost every imaginable type of illness and injury.

Dr. Chow is licensed to practice medicine in Illinois, Georgia, and New York, and regularly shuttles back and forth between New York and Chicago. He is the founder, CEO, and president of multispecialty clinics offering integrative medicine and diverse treatment modalities. The clinic in Chicago was originally named Hakuju. Now renamed Nippon Clinics, they are located in Chicago, Atlanta, San Diego, and New York. In 1996, Dr. Chow helped set up an American-style clinic in Beijing, China.

Dr. Chow contributes frequently to numerous newspapers and magazines, including *U.S. Frontline* and *Yomiuri*. He has appeared on television and his practice has been featured in newspapers and magazines, including *Asia.*

Dr. Chow is a member of American Academy of Emergency Medicine; American Academy of Physician Executives; American Academy of Sports Medicine; American Academy of General Medicine; American Academy of Family Practice; Nippon Industrial Medicine Association; American Japanese Physicians Association. Having too much time on his hands, Dr. Chow has recently created a medical software company, Atomu Systems LLC. Dr. Chow is known among his friends and associates for his unbounded energy, personal warmth, and sense of humor — had he not become a medical doctor, he could undoubtedly have become a comedian.

Dedication

We dedicate this book to our mother, who has inspired us with her indomitable spirit. Late in life she became a published novelist and essayist (with fan mail from all over the world) and blossomed from chronic illness into an amazingly strong and healthy individual. Always young at heart, most of her friends are half her age.

This book is also dedicated to our father without whose foresight and financial support (lots of it!) neither of us would have been blessed with the education and career opportunities that we had. Cheryl in particular thanks him for his help while she was too ill to work full time.

Acknowledgments

I would like to thank everyone, especially various health care practitioners, whose knowledge, expertise, and experience helped shape this book.

Much gratitude goes to my friends Sandra Whitefield, MSW, LCSW; Melanie Hecht, tech writer-chiropractor-real estate investor; Ann Worth, activist for workers' rights and my partner in crime from grade school; Charmaine Getz, writer/editor; Jane Mack Cozzo, writer/university instructor; and Amy Pasley, C.M.T., for their support and encouragement throughout the writing of this book.

I would like to express my appreciation to my brother and coauthor, Dr. James Chow, not only for his share of the work, but for all the great restaurants he takes me to whenever I go to New York or Chicago. I'll make sure I visit him more often.

Special thanks to Natasha Graf for coming up with the idea for this book and painstakingly reviewing the outlines, and to my editor Tonya Cupp. Her help and support, and the help of her editorial assistants, made the writing of *Hypoglycemia For Dummies* go much more smoothly than it would have otherwise.

Thanks to all our technical editors, especially Dr. Iljong Kim, for his invaluable input and for putting up with so many questions from me. I'd also like to acknowledge recipe editor Emily Nolan for her conscientious work.

Last — and certainly least — I'd like to acknowledge my cat Saki for the reality check she's so kindly given me by periodically barfing on my manuscript.

Publisher's Acknowledgments

We're proud of this book; please send us your comments through our Dummies online registration form located at www.dummies.com/register/.

Some of the people who helped bring this book to market include the following:

Acquisitions, Editorial, and Media Development

Project Editor: Tonya Maddox Cupp

Acquisitions Editor: Tracy Boggier

Copy Editor: Greg Pearson

Acquisitions Coordinator: Holly Grimes

Technical Editor: Martin Graf, M.D.

Editorial Manager: Jennifer Ehrlich

Editorial Assistant: Elizabeth Rea

Cartoons: Rich Tennant, www.the5thwave.com

Production

Project Coordinator: Maridee Ennis

Layout and Graphics: Seth Conley, Stephanie Jumper, Michael Kruzil, Kristin McMullan, Tiffany Muth, Janet Seib, Julie Trippetti, Jeremy Unger

Proofreaders: Tyler Connoley, Dave Faust, Susan Moritz, Angel Perez, TECHBOOKS Production Services

Indexer: TECHBOOKS Production Services

Publishing and Editorial for Consumer Dummies

    Diane Graves Steele, Vice President and Publisher, Consumer Dummies

    Joyce Pepple, Acquisitions Director, Consumer Dummies

    Kristin A. Cocks, Product Development Director, Consumer Dummies

    Michael Spring, Vice President and Publisher, Travel

    Brice Gosnell, Publishing Director, Travel

    Suzanne Jannetta, Editorial Director, Travel

Publishing for Technology Dummies

    Andy Cummings, Vice President and Publisher, Dummies Technology/General User

Composition Services

    Gerry Fahey, Vice President of Production Services

    Debbie Stailey, Director of Composition Services

Contents at a Glance

Table of Contents

Introduction

● ●

*I*f you pick up this book, chances are that you've been suffering from the blues for a long time: the low blood sugar blues, that is. If you're hypoglycemic, you know that you don't have to go to an amusement park to experience the roller coaster effect; your blood sugar does it for you automatically, thank you very much. In addition, you may get the jitters often, especially after a stretch of time without food; you're nervous, edgy, and irritable. You're chronically tired, and you wake up in the morning not feeling the least bit rested. Or maybe you have other complaints, such as depression, that just don't respond to medical treatments — or any other remedies.

Your colleagues, friends, and family may be tired of your moods, your chronic fatigue, and your various aches and illnesses, none of which seems to have a clear, attributable cause. You've been to many doctors. And what do they tell you? They tell you that all the lab tests have come out "essentially negative." You're afraid that the doctors regard you as neurotic or, at best, a hypochondriac. Or perhaps you received a clear diagnosis. But now your real struggles begin. No magic pills can instantly cure you.

The good news is that, with a better understanding of hypoglycemia and the program of recovery outlined in this book, you can regain your health, your wits, and your sense of humor. And who knows, you may — depending on your genes and, aside from hypoglycemia, whatever else may be going on with your body — appreciate life more than many of your healthier brethren that you now envy.

About This Book

We have good news for you busy people! You don't have to read this book from cover to cover. You can turn to the section that seems most relevant to you and start reading. If you suspect that someone close to you is hypoglycemic, you may want to start with Chapter 14 and go from there.

Conventions Used in This Book

To make everything as easy as possible, all medical terms have been italicized and explained immediately — you don't even have to flip to a glossary to find out what they mean. We've also attempted to explain any other words or concepts that may be difficult to understand or may be subject to misunderstanding.

Whenever we mention hypoglycemia in this book, unless otherwise indicated (and we'll make that amply clear), we're talking about the hypoglycemia that's related to one's diet — the type that people are normally talking about when they complain about feeling weak from low blood sugar.

We're using the word *recovery* because health is an ongoing process, not something that you can attain with a quick-fix approach to life. Your challenge is to correct not only the imbalances of your body but also the way you live, work, play, and relate to others.

By the way, the *we* in this book isn't a royal *we* (as in, we're just so much better than the average person, that we can tell you how everyone thinks) but a plural *we* that refers to the two co-authors writing this book, Cheryl and Jim (Dr. Chow).

Icons Used in This Book

The icons are signposts to help you identify what parts are indispensable and what parts may be interesting but can be skipped without fear.

This icon presents very important information that you should be aware of. Don't ignore this icon! Doing so may be detrimental.

Just do like the icon says and everybody'll be fine. The book has a lot of information, but this icon highlights the stuff that'll do you good.

This icon marks paragraphs that contain technical or medical terms.

This icon indicates useful information about hypoglycemia. It can save you time, or money, if you're lucky.

Foolish Assumptions

If you pick up this book, we assume that you

- ✔ Suffer from symptoms associated with hypoglycemia (or someone close to you suffers from the symptoms).

- ✔ Are not a specialist in the medical field (You won't be flummoxed by technical terms that aren't clearly explained, or concepts that are hard to follow.)

- ✔ Are aware of the controversy surrounding this syndrome but accept — or at least suspect — that such a medical problem indeed exists.

How This Book Is Organized

This book is divided into six parts to make it easier for you to navigate through all the material it contains. It's designed to be a handy reference for the busy person, as much of the relevant information has been compiled together under one cover for your convenience.

Part 1: Addressing Your Ups And Downs: Could This Be Hypoglycemia?

Part I addresses all the most important facts about hypoglycemia. What causes it? Who's most susceptible? This part talks about some of the hypoglycemic complications that may result from diabetes, as well as about other common occurrences that you should watch out for.

Part II: Getting A Diagnosis: Do I Or Don't I?

Perhaps it was a chance remark or something you read; you have some cause to suspect that you or your loved ones may be hypoglycemic. This part helps you determine if you suffer from this condition. We help you sort through all the complexities and permutations of this syndrome and rule out other possible causes for what's ailing you.

Part III: Getting Off Your Bleached-Flour Buns and Treating the Problem

Food. It's everyone's favorite subject. Here we discuss the role of nutrition in health (bear with us, we try to make it as fun as a stroll in the park) and, in particular, the great significance it has for the hypoglycemic person. We discuss the underlying biochemical disorder in chronic hypoglycemia. If you have hypoglycemia, you have to change your eating habits. We let you know why.

Part IV: Emulating Lifestyles of the Well and Healthy

We map out the lifestyle that will help you achieve the vibrant health you desire. We chart a course through the two indispensable pillars that provide a solid foundation for health: diet and exercise. We show you how to create a practical diet that works for you and explore how to choose exercises that are fun for you.

Part V: Spinning a Network of Support for Yourself

Everyone needs the support of other people from time to time; none of us can make it completely alone. In this part, we show you how to set up a support network.

Part VI: The Part of Tens

You want some more help? You got it — from both this part and the resources it directs you to.

Where to Go from Here

You don't have to read from cover to cover. Where should you go?

- ✔ You know nothing about hypoglycemia: Chapter 2 can give you the nitty gritty technical scoop.
- ✔ You know you have to eat right to get through this thing, but you don't know where to start: Chapter 6 can get you going, and Chapter 17 can help, too.
- ✔ You're hungry: Recipes abound in Chapter 15.

Part I

Addressing Your Ups and Downs: Could This Be Hypoglycemia?

The 5th Wave
By Rich Tennant

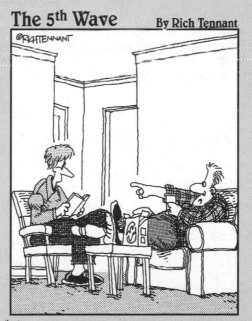

"C'mon, Darrel! Someone with hypoglycemia shouldn't be lying around all day. Whereas someone with no life, like myself, has a very good reason."

In this part . . .

If you want to know the most important facts about hypoglycemia, you can find them here. This part lists the different types of hypoglycemia that are known to the medical world. We cover some of the hypoglycemic complications that can result from diabetes, and we tell you about other common conditions that you should watch out for. We also show you just how many symptoms are associated with hypoglycemia.

Chapter 1

Riding the Blood Sugar Roller Coaster Isn't Any Fun

In This Chapter

▶ Defining hypoglycemia

▶ Linking hypoglycemia and diabetes

▶ Identifying symptoms of hypoglycemia

▶ Looking at who's prone to blood sugar imbalance

▶ Taking the road to radiant health

Defining hypoglycemia is easy. It's low *(hypo)* blood sugar *(glycemia)*. Modern medicine, which is Western medicine as it's practiced in developed countries, recognizes two major categories of hypoglycemia:

✔ **Organic hypoglycemia:** This type, which is very rare, is caused by glandular defects or tumors.

✔ **Functional hypoglycemia:** This type of hypoglycemia typically occurs because of an imbalance in the body chemistry, probably due to an overactive pancreas producing too much insulin.

• *Fasting hypoglycemia* is sometimes classified as being part of functional hypoglycemia. This type of hypoglycemia can occur when you haven't eaten for a while. How long that is depends on the individual, but it's generally several hours after a meal.

• *Idiopathic reactive hypoglycemia,* or simply *reactive hypoglycemia,* is the most common type of functional hypoglycemia. "Idiopathic" is just a fancy word that doctors use to say, "We haven't got a clue what causes it." (Now you know how to profess ignorance and still sound smart!) "Reactive" relates to how your body responds to the food you eat.

If you're suffering from idiopathic reactive hypoglycemia, your body generally reacts negatively to sugar and simple starches, because it can't handle the excess sugar load. You usually start feeling the effect about 2 to 4 hours after eating "bad" foods.

Western medicine recognizes organic and fasting hypoglycemia, which both generally have clear-cut causes, as legitimate. What's controversial, however, is the diagnosis of reactive hypoglycemia. This is the type of hypoglycemia that people are referring to when they complain of being hypoglycemic. Reactive hypoglycemia is also this book's focus. In the rest of this book, unless otherwise stated, we're talking about reactive hypoglycemia.

Okay, now that we have the definitions out of the way, buckle down. This book takes you on a special tour of a condition that's actually more common than people realize. You can find out if you're susceptible, how hypoglycemia is linked to diabetes, and the symptoms you should watch for. The good news is that you're not stuck on a merry-go-round. This chapter — and the rest of the book — gives you all the tools you need to address and control hypoglycemia.

Like a Greased Pig: Easy to Define, Tough to Pin Down

Well, if your blood sugar level is low, you obviously have a low-blood sugar condition! Because hypoglycemia is so easy to define, you'd think that determining who has low blood sugar would be a simple matter. All you should have to do is measure the blood sugar and *voilà!* — you have inconvertible proof that someone has hypoglycemia.

Alas, it's not that cut and dried. Experts disagree on what constitutes a hypoglycemic condition. Today's standard medical practice is to consider hypoglycemic levels of blood sugar lower than 45 milligrams per deciliter of blood. The benchmark used to be higher, but it has shifted downwards over the years, and doctors still disagree with one another in terms of finding and diagnosing the condition. For instance, some health practitioners argue *no* range of blood sugar is definitive in determining hypoglycemia; they believe instead that the speed in which the blood sugar drops is more important than how low it goes. (Chapter 4 gives you more detailed information about diagnoses and measurements.)

And that's not the only controversy surrounding hypoglycemia. These bits add to the trouble:

- ✔ Syptoms are nonspecific. (You can read more in Chapter 3).

- ✔ Symptoms don't always correlate with blood glucose (sugar) concentrations measured during an oral glucose test. (More on this in Chapter 4.)

- ✔ Glucose levels are rarely measured when people develop symptoms spontaneously (not easy to manage unless someone follows them around with a syringe).

- ✔ Hypoglycemia is a misnomer. Rather than low blood sugar, it's more a matter of the body being unable to effectively absorb certain carbohydrates. Different people react differently to ingested sugars and carbohydrates, with some having a higher tolerance level than others. Thus, the condition may be better described as *carbohydrate intolerance* or *glucose instability syndrome*.

In the 1970s, after several books popularized hypoglycemia, many people jumped on the hypoglycemia bandwagon, and it became an over-diagnosed condition — a fad disease that most respectable health care practitioners strived to steer clear of. So it's understandable that many doctors are skeptical. It's also unfortunate, because they're unable to help patients who ask "If I'm so healthy, why do I feel so bad?"

Identifying key symptoms

The symptoms aren't fatal, but they can seriously detract from the quality of life. The immediate physical symptoms of low blood sugar are

- ✔ Mental confusion (brain fog)
- ✔ Inability to think rationally
- ✔ Weakness
- ✔ Shakiness

These symptoms can be alleviated by eating. The more debilitating symptoms of chronic hypoglycemia, however, are longer lasting and not immediately relieved by eating. Chapter 3 talks more about symptoms, and Part IV addresses some of the most prevailing and consuming symptoms, such as depression.

And so the link between food and symptoms is undeniable. Face food facts! This book can help you do that by offering alternatives to the foods you currently eat. Flip to Chapter 6 for info on the foods you can and can't safely eat as a hypoglycemic. Go to the

Cheat Sheet for tips on how to deal with foods you shouldn't have but that call out to you when you're at your weakest. If you have a partner and/or children, flip to Chapter 13 for help on setting up a diet lifestyle with your family.

Arriving at a diagnosis

Some people may have low blood sugar levels without hypoglycemic symptoms, while others may have symptoms of hypoglycemia, even severe ones, even though their blood sugar is within normal range. Therefore, measuring blood sugar is an unreliable way to diagnose hypoglycemia. For these and other reasons, hypoglycemia is often dismissed as imaginary. Despite the protests of some medical organizations, many nutritionally oriented MDs, naturopaths, and other alternative practitioners claim that hypoglycemia is a real clinical entity, and they have successfully treated the disorder by changing their patients' diets. You can read more about these medical practitioners in Chapter 5.

The best way to diagnose the disorder is through a combination of various lab tests (discussed in detail in Chapter 4) and an assessment of symptoms (discussed in Chapters 3 and 4). In addition, you can try eliminating foods from your diet (see Chapter 4) to see if symptoms clear up. The food journal discussed in Chapter 6 can also help you determine which foods may affect you.

You should see a doctor before you do anything, especially if it's been several years since your last physical checkup.

Knowing Who's Prone

Hypoglycemia can strike anyone at any age. Unlike diabetes, not enough studies have been performed to create an accurate profile. Nevertheless, because reactive hypoglycemia can be an early sign of diabetes, it's reasonable to believe that hypoglycemics and diabetics share a genetic predisposition for metabolic disorders and similar risks for environmental triggers.

Research suggests that the following people are hypoglycemia's likeliest victims:

- ✔ Women suffering from premenstrual syndrome (PMS).
- ✔ People suffering from severe stress.

> ✔ People who are overweight (though some are underweight due to their faulty carbohydrate metabolism).
>
> ✔ Alcoholics. Some researchers have concluded that alcoholism is actually an unrecognized problem with body chemistry, and that all alcoholics are, in fact, hypoglycemics.

Prevailing problem: The pudge!

The sugar and refined carbohydrate-laden diet that the majority of people in developed countries eat has led to a host of health problems, with hypoglycemia being one of them.

Although most medical and health organizations recommend that no more than 10 percent of total caloric intake be derived from the refined sugars added to foods, the fact is that most people in developed countries eat far more than that (possibly three times that amount). And what's even more alarming is that some lesser-developed Asian countries are getting a sweet tooth that rivals the richer nations! Statistics show that the consumption of sugar worldwide is increasing by 1 to 2 percent every year. Small wonder so many people have a pudge of a problem.

Like a couple of hooligans: Linking hypoglycemia and diabetes

You probably know someone who has diabetes. But you may not know that hypoglycemia and diabetes are linked. Blood sugar imbalance underlies both disorders. In the case of hypoglycemics, experts theorize that over a prolonged period of time, too much insulin (from eating sugar and simple starches) followed by a blood sugar drop results in cells losing their sensitivity to insulin. Thus, hypoglycemia is considered to be a pre-diabetic condition.

Both diabetics and hypoglycemics should treat their condition through dietary means. The recommended diet for diabetes and hypoglycemia is, in fact, quite similar — although low-blood-sugar sufferers are often advised to reduce their carbohydrate intake, at least during the early part of treatment. Chapter 3 gives more information about diabetes and hypoglycemia and how they're related. Chapter 6 gives the scoop about using your diet to your health's advantage.

Heading Towards Better Health

A paradigm shift has been taking place in recent years in most Western countries, as more people are searching for alternative practices for attaining good health — something that crisis-driven Western medicine is unable to offer. The new paradigm holds a high regard for the nutritional basis of disease. The new paradigm, with its holistic, body-mind approach to health and healing, can more fully address hypoglycemia's spectrum of problems. A *holistic* approach looks at the patient's entire lifestyle, in addition to diet, for clues to what's causing the illness. (Part IV shows you how to take a holistic approach to your health. For a broader view of this lifestyle, check out Wiley Publishing's *Mind-Body Fitness For Dummies*.)

Think of this as a journey toward greater health — a journey of transformation, moving from the way you've been to a new approach to living and a greater sense of well-being. In this book, we show you how the transition into a healthy life can be smooth and not as painful as you may suspect.

The following list shows where you may be starting. If you follow the physical and food advice given in this book, you'll come out on the other side looking and feeling a whole lot better.

- ✔ **Not eating right — right now.** You should be eating six small meals, or three small meals and three light snacks, per day, though you may eat more frequently if you need to when you first embark on the program. This diet is very similar to a diabetic diet and doesn't include sweets or sugars.

    Chapter 15 gives you recipes for a hypoglycemically-correct diet; Chapter 6 gives dietary details. You can safely follow any recipes created for diabetics as long as you refrain from using artificial sweeteners. The Internet is a great source for healthy recipes. Plenty of good diabetes cookbooks exist as well, including the *Diabetic Cookbook For Dummies* (Wiley Publishing).

- ✔ **Overweight.** For various reasons, low blood sugar can lead to weight gain. One reason is that you may be giving in to an increased desire for sweets; Chapter 8 can help get you motivated to get moving. In addition, overeating sweets and starches overstimulates insulin production, and too much insulin causes excess storage of fat.

- ✔ **Underweight.** You may have been gorging yourself on sugars and starches in a futile attempt to gain weight. (And evoking jealousy among your friends in the process.) If so, addressing your underlying metabolism disorder can help you put on the pounds that you want and need.

✔ **Combating depression and mood disorders.** When Abraham Lincoln said, "People are as happy as they make up their minds to be," little knowledge existed about the basics of depression. (Ironically, evidence suggests that Lincoln himself was a generally depressed person, who never did fully "make up his mind" to be happy. Could he have suffered from hypoglycemia?)

Even today, the common knowledge and perception of the nature of depression lags behind discoveries. Well-intentioned people may try to convince a depressed person to "snap out of it." If you're on the receiving end of this advice, it can be devastating. You end up feeling blamed for being whiny, hopeless, and helpless, knowing all too well that the solution isn't that simple. Chronic depression is a mental disorder that isn't necessarily precipitated by life events. Chapter 10 talks about this topic in depth.

✔ **Lacking a solid support structure.** When you have a condition that undermines your effectiveness in daily life and chips away at your confidence and self-esteem, you need a bridge. That bridge must have a strong foundation to help you get from where you are today to where you want to be. The support structure that you create for yourself is this bridge. (See? It's all up to you: Not only are you responsible for food and exercise, but finding support is all about you, too.)

A support person or group can help guide you through, especially when you're just beginning your recovery program. Chapter 11 tells you how to get the support you need, and Chapter 17 shows resources that can help you. Chapters 13 and 14 talk about more intimate relationships and how to gain — and give! — support in them.

Every individual is so different that predicting a time frame of recovery is difficult, but in general, you should start to see a noticeable improvement in your health in about three months. Having an occasional bad food day won't negate your progress — but don't kid yourself. Going off your food plan for several days, not to mention weeks, will definitely impede your progress.

Chapter 2

Flipping Through the Hypoglycemia Catalog

· ·

· ·

In this chapter, we don't rhapsodize about the marvel of engineering that is the human body. We tell it like it is so that you know the hormonal basics that take place whenever you chow down. That way you can understand why diet is the cornerstone of treatment for hypoglycemics.

Digesting Some Physical Food

Generally, a meal provides nutrients that reach your body over a span of about four hours. However, your cells demand nutrients around the clock. (They were the first ones to demand 24/7 service.)

Digestion begins in your mouth — this is why your parents and other well-meaning people tell you to chew your food — and continues in your stomach. The food has to be broken down before the nutrients can be used. It's a complex process that can be quite a mouthful to describe in just a few words. So we break down the steps for you to help you better digest the information.

Breaking down proteins

G'head, take a bite:

1. **Saliva comes into contact with food.**

   It's the salivary enzymes in the mouth that partially break down some of the starch into a simple sugar called glucose. *Glucose* is the sugar in your blood stream; it's also your body's energy source.

2. **Your body recognizes any alien proteins and breaks them down into basic amino acids.**

   Amino acids are molecular units that make up all proteins. For an example of an alien protein, think of steak. Steak is composed of protein, carbohydrates, and fat. The protein in the steak is in the form of beef protein, which doesn't do you a whole lot of good if you're a homo sapien. (We presume you are, because you're reading this book, but if you're not — well, we've heard of stranger things!) Why? Because it's got to be converted into human protein before your body can use it.

3. **Your body reconstructs some of the amino acids into human protein.**

   That protein is now available for growth, repair, and other vital physical functions.

4. **Some of the amino acids become human carbohydrates, which are converted into basic sugars: glycogen and glucose.**

   Glycogen is the sugar your body stores, mostly in the liver but also in muscle tissue. Hundreds of branches stick out from glycogen, and on each brach is a glucose, which is attached to the next glucose. All are readily accessible to the glycogen-splitting enzymes.

   Excess glucose is converted to glycogen or fatty acids. If you're in the fasting state, however, the triacylglycerols and amino acids produce glucose. Glycogen is not produced.

5. **The liver converts some of the excess energy into fat.**

   Excess fat gets stored in the fat cells to meet long-term energy needs.

Pancreas

Now it's time for the pancreas to play its part. The *pancreas* is an organ that

- Manufactures *enzymes* to digest food
- Manufactures *bicarbonate* to neutralize stomach acid
- Manufactures *glucagon,* a protein hormone that stimulates the release of glucose into the blood
- Secretes *insulin* when alerted that you're eating carbs (Insulin is a powerful hormone that, among other things, chaperones the glucose to the body's cells, instructing the cells to take in the glucose. That's critical, because glucose is your body's fuel.)

Carbohydrates are basically chains of sugar molecules. The carbs you eat are mostly chains of glucose molecules. The shorter the chain, the sweeter the taste. Some chains are longer and more complicated, having many links and even branches. Hence, short chains are known as *simple carbohydrates,* and longer ones as *complex carbohydrates.* Simple or complex, carbs are composed entirely of sugar.

If the blood delivers more glucose than the cells can take in, the liver and muscles take up the surplus.

- The muscles hog two-thirds of the body's total store of glucose.
- The liver stores the other third and makes it available when the brain or other organs need to draw on the supply.

Here's how the pancreas helps regulate your blood sugar level:

1. **You eat a meal and insulin becomes the dominant hormone in your body.**

2. **Insulin is suppressed four to six hours later when glucagon shows up.**

    This happens as your metabolism shifts gears. Glucagon suppresses insulin by releasing glucose into the blood.

    - When blood glucose levels drop too low, the pancreas releases glucagon.

    - Suppression of the insulin allows the liver to release glucose.

3. **As long as the blood glucose levels are within normal range, insulin regulates glucose metabolism.**

   If the blood glucose level dips too low, *counterregulatory hormones* (hormones that oppose insulin's action) are released.

Insulin stores the glucose in the liver and muscle cells, and glucagon removes it from storage as needed.

Insulin gone awry

In order for your body's check-and-balance mechanism to work properly, the demand for insulin must subside at times. Assume this nasty scenario:

1. **You repeatedly chow down on snacks high in sugar and starch.**

2. **Your body has to constantly pump out insulin.**

3. **Too much insulin!**

4. **The insulin receptors on the cells lose some of their sensitivity.**

5. **The pancreas secretes more insulin, hoping to get the receptors to respond.**

6. **Way too much insulin!**

7. **Insulin rounds up the glucose from the blood stream and drives it into the cells.**

   The result is *hypoglycemia,* or low blood sugar. (Doctors who don't believe that hypoglycemia exists in so-called healthy people — in other words, non-diabetic people — would argue that hypoglycemia can't occur as just described.)

8. **The insulin receptors become desensitized, and insulin can't deliver enough glucose into the cells.**

   The result is a condition known as insulin resistance. See Chapter 4 for more on this condition and its link to hypoglycemia.

9. **Eventually, more sugar remains in the bloodstream.**

   The result is type 2 diabetes.

This is an admittedly oversimplified picture and just one scenario that can cause hypoglycemia in people who are genetically susceptible.

The point to remember is that when a person who's sensitive to carbohydrates (see Chapter 4 for more about carbohydrate sensitivity) eats carbs, the blood sugar increases more rapidly than it should. This situation results in a rapid rise and fall in both insulin and blood sugar levels.

Bear in mind that carbohydrates only make up part of the foods that directly affect blood sugar levels. Protein and fats are slowly absorbed, so the sensitive insulin apparatus is less likely to be triggered. Thus, small, regular meals consisting of protein or fats and some carbs keep the blood sugar stabilized, preventing sudden rises and falls in glucose.

Now you can appreciate what a complex dance the chemicals and hormones have to perform in order to keep your blood sugar level within a narrow range. The picture isn't yet complete, however. There are more dancers and more steps to the process, as you see later in this chapter.

Tracing Cause and Effect

Hypoglycemia has many causes, some of which aren't related to what you eat, but we don't spend too much time on them. (Our editor wants only info that you can actually use. What a novel idea!)

Just remember that hypoglycemia treatment depends totally on the underlying medical illnesses. So go see your doctor first — don't diagnose yourself!

Multiple causes

People often suffer from many of the symptoms of hypoglycemia even when their blood sugar isn't particularly low. The term *pseudohypoglycemia* refers to the symptoms of hypoglycemia that occur without low blood sugar.

It's a matter of debate, but most doctors argue that hypoglycemia doesn't occur without an underlying medical illness that's unrelated to what you eat. (Chapter 4 talks about this more.) When there are no organic causes for hypoglycemia, the hormone epinephrine (adrenaline) is likely involved. It appears that insulin can stimulate epinephrine release in some sensitive people.

In some patients, low blood sugar occurs mainly because of a defect in glucose production, while in others, the problem is the result of an excessive use of glucose. Sometimes the low blood sugar level is the result of both reasons. Other causes of hypo-glycemia are profound malnutrition, prolonged exercise, chronic renal failure, late pregnancy, severe liver deficiency, and liver diseases, such as viral hepatitis or cirrhosis.

Exhausting your adrenals

It's 11 p.m. Do you know where your adrenals are? Hopefully they're tucked away all safe and sound in bed. Seriously, if you replied that the adrenals are located above your kidneys, you're absolutely correct. The *adrenals,* which are no bigger than a walnut, rise up kind of like mushrooms from the top of each kidney and are intimately involved with normal blood sugar regulation — very important for the hypoglycemically challenged person.

The hormones these little guys secrete influence all the major physiological process in the body. For starters, they affect how carbs and fats are utilized, how fats and proteins are converted into energy, and how stored fat is distributed. (Remember that the next time you're in a bathing suit.)

1. **You bounce the mortgage check, one of the kids gets the flu, and the cat barfs on your new bedspread.**

   Now that's what we call stress. (Or your average Monday.)

2. **Your adrenals work too hard and become fatigued from too much stress.**

   The adrenals react to any situation that they believe to be an emergency by secreting the hormone *adrenaline.* In the not-so-good-old-days, the fight-or-flight response was triggered when a neanderthal man saw a rabid buffalo charging at him. More adrenaline was pumped into his bloodstream to get him ready to either fight the creature or flee. (Feet, don't fail me now!) Today an emergency is more likely to be a car that cuts in front of you, a boss who gives you a dressing down, or a customer who calls you names.

3. **Cortisol levels drop lower than normal.**

   The adrenal hormone *cortisol* keeps blood sugar at adequate levels. A low level of cortisol makes it tough for your body to maintain normal blood sugar levels. If your adrenals are sluggish, your liver will be slow to convert glycogen to glucose. Normally, fats, proteins, and carbs can be converted into glucose, but this process is more difficult when the adrenals are fatigued. In this situation, one of the blood sugar glitches can arise.

4. **Your liver has difficulty converting glycogen back to glucose.**

   Glycogen, or stored sugar, has to be converted into *glucose* (blood sugar) before the body can use it. When your liver has difficulty converting glycogen to glucose, less blood sugar is available and your brain is deprived of fuel. When your brain isn't getting enough sugar, you can develop hypoglycemic symptoms, such as lightheadedness and disorientation.

Ravaging your health: The couch and the potato

We've been programmed to think that carbohydrates are not only delectable but good for you. Yet, even complex carbohydrates like whole grains can be problematic if your body doesn't metabolize carbs properly.

Burp. You've eaten your fill; you're stuffed to the gill. You're lying contentedly on the couch, remote in hand, relaxing after a hard day of work. Well, you may be at rest, but check this out:

1. **Your digestive tract is busier than the pizza man. It's delivering glucose to the bloodstream.**

2. **The blood carries this glucose to your liver.**

3. **The liver breaks the glucose down into small fragments and puts them together into the more permanent energy storage compound — in other words, fat.**

4. **The fat is released into the blood, carried to the body's fatty tissues, and deposited there.**

   Unlike the liver cells, which can store only about half a day's supply of glycogen, the fat cells — much to the chagrin of dieters — can store unlimited quantities of fat.

You can find out how fast carbs become glucose and enter the bloodstream by checking out the *glycemic index (GI)* of food. (See Chapter 6 for more on this topic.)

TIP

Sugar by any other name is just as deadly

Did you know that Elizabeth I had black teeth because of her sugar craving? Just thought we'd throw that in.

You should be aware that products can be called sugar-free if they don't contain common table sugar (sucrose). Even if they don't have sucrose, they still may contain a fair amount of sugars that can spike your blood sugar. So read labels carefully. Any ingredients ending with "-ose" are actually just a form of sugar. Better avoid them.

Sugar, sugar, everywhere — except where you need it

Sugar. Honey. Sweetie-pie. Terms of endearment reflect the desirability of sweet tastes.

Sugar is surprisingly prevalent in dishes you may least suspect: soups, cured meats, salad dressings, and sauces, for example. One tablespoon of regular ketchup contains a teaspoon of sugar. Hoisin sauce, which used in Chinese cooking, has just as much sugar, if not more. A can of soda pop contains several tablespoons of sugar. Even diet foods contain large amounts of rapidly acting carbohydrates or alternative sweeteners like aspartame (which has been linked to cancer).

If we're surrounded by sugar, how can anyone possibly be suffering from low blood sugar? That's precisely the point. Because everything is so sugar-laden, keeping a steady level of blood sugar has become difficult. Just because someone is suffering from low blood sugar, it doesn't mean that she should eat sugar. This statement may, at first, appear to be a contradiction. The paradox is that the more sugar you eat, the less sugar you have in your blood.

The blood sugar that your body needs to function can be obtained easily through unrefined carbs, protein, and fats. The truth is that even if you eat absolutely no glucose or refined sugar, you'll still have plenty of blood sugar as long as your body is functioning properly. Chapter 6 explains why refined carbs are harmful but unrefined carbs are okay.

Addressing Food Addictions

A sweet link may exist between various forms of addictions and low blood sugar. The connection may lie in feel-good hormones called *beta-endorphins,* which are produced in the *opiod system,* the reward pathway of the brain. Scientists are now working with the hypothesis that the presence of beta-endorphins in the reward pathway regions in the brain is key to the development of addiction to opiods like heroin. Beta-endorphins give you a feeling of euphoria, or a sense of being on top of the world.

Not surprisingly, other things can offer such addictive relationships to varying degrees.

- **Saying sayonara to the sauce.** The fact is, alcohol is a simple carb that's rapidly converted into sugar. It creates an addictive high that's quickly followed by a low. Hypoglycemia in alcoholics usually occurs after a several-day alcohol binge or in a malnourished state, which causes glycogen depletion in the liver and blocks glucose synthesis.

  Most treatment programs emphasize psychological factors and neglect possible biochemical deficiencies and body chemistry. Many problems attributed to an alcoholic's personality or life history may actually be caused by faulty body chemistry. If you're working toward a recovery from drinking, try addressing both your body (with dietary changes like those suggested in Chapter 6) and your mind (with support from groups like AA).

- **Conquering the carb crave.** Always craving the carbo rush? If so, you may be
  - Not getting enough protein
  - Seeing an early warning sign that your stress level is too high (Chapter 9 shows you how to lower the boom on stress.)
  - eating an out-of-balance diet
  - unconsciously using self-medication to lift your mood

  Chapter 6 offers more detailed information about carbs.

- **Kicking caffeine in the coffeemaker.** Caffeine has an effect similar to sugar, although the results may not be so immediate. It triggers the release of stored glycogen to temporarily increase the blood sugar level. Chapter 13 offers ideas on how to kick your addiction to caffeine.

✔ **Knocking out nicotine.** Enough has been said about the bad effects of cigarettes and other tobacco products. But are you aware of the effect that nicotine has on blood sugar? Light up a cigarette, and ping! You just boosted your blood sugar. You suddenly feel euphoric. Why? Because nicotine stimulates the adrenal glands. Unfortunately, smoking creates a desire for caffeine, sweet foods, and alcohol.

Start by adjusting your diet and taking the necessary supplements (which are described in Chapter 7). Hypnosis, meditation, and breathing techniques may also help (and some are described in Chapter 9). If you continue to smoke, even if you follow the correct diet, you may not notice an improvement in symptoms because adrenal stimulation from the nicotine is constantly triggering the release of glucose into the blood — and the sugar spike is rapidly followed by a crash.

Chapter 3

Symptoms without a Cause

● ●

In This Chapter

▶ Recognizing the symptoms of chronic hypoglycemia

▶ Discovering the hidden causes of hypoglycemia

▶ Examining the link between hypoglycemia and diabetes

● ●

*H*aving hypoglycemia is certainly *not* more fun than a barrel
full of monkeys — but sometimes it may feel like you have
monkeys running around, keeping your mind edgy and unfocused.
At times you may feel cold, anxious, or nervous; or you may be so
down and depressed that you're virtually digging in the ditches. (If
that's the case, check out Chapter 10.) Then, before you know it,
your heart is racing so fast that you'd think you were running from
a herd of elephants. Meanwhile, you're experiencing memory loss;
it's getting so that you can't remember what you've forgotten.

If you often experience these symptoms, you may have chronic
hypoglycemia. Or not. Determining whether you have this disorder
can be downright confusing, because the symptoms mimic so many
other illnesses. This chapter clarifies the muddy waters. (For information about getting a proper medical diagnosis from a doctor,
turn to Chapter 4.) At the same time, this chapter makes clear the
connection between diabetes and hypoglycemia. Chapter 2 also
discusses the hypo-diabetes link if you want to know even more.

Jumping on Stage: No, You're Not Faking It

Nothing's clear cut about hypoglycemia. Why would its stages be
any different? Generally speaking, doctors can detect two basic
stages. Each stage can last anywhere from weeks to years, depending on the individual and the underlying cause.

✔ **Stage 1:** Depression, fatigue, lethargy, poor concentration, and memory loss

✔ **Stage 2:** Agitation, fast heart beat, cold and clammy hands, and possibly full-blown panic attacks

That's the fun part. The not-so-fun part is that most people are going to label you a hypochondriac. As far as they're concerned, the problem's all in your mind. And no wonder, hypoglycemia has just too many darn symptoms. (For more information on talking about the disorder with those you know and love, check out Chapters 13 and 14.) When confronted with the long list of nonspecific complaints that hypoglycemics generally present, many doctors may be tempted to dismiss it as hogwash. (That's the medical term for "I'd rather scrub Porky Pig in a tub than deal with this.") Don't let the doctor's diagnosis deter you. Find a doctor or health care practitioner who truly understands hypoglycemia. See Chapter 5 for some good ways to find one.

If you suspect that you may have hypoglycemia, get a proper check-up to rule out other causes. The kind of chronic hypoglycemia we talk about in this book may be disabling, but it's not fatal. If something else is causing your low blood sugar, you can end up harming yourself by not getting proper treatment. (See "Unmasking Hypoglycemia's Hidden Faces" later in this chapter for various causes of hypoglycemia.)

Odd, You Have a Puny Bod: Physical Symptoms

If you're like most people with hypoglycemia, you wake up feeling tired and exhausted, and your body may feel achy. You may not feel too good in the morning, but you often start to feel much better in the evening. (Generally, people have higher levels of blood sugar in the evening.)

The long and short of it is that there's a long list of physical symptoms classically attributed to hypoglycemia. When checking out this list, look for a group of symptoms that *persist over time*.

Here are just some of the symptoms associated with hypoglycemia:

- Accident prone
- Aching eye sockets
- Backache and muscle pain
- Bad breath
- Blurred vision
- Chatterbox (talking a lot)
- Chronically cold hands and feet
- Convulsions
- Dizziness
- Drowsiness
- Fainting or blackouts
- Family history of diabetes or low blood sugar
- Fatigue or exhaustion
- Headaches
- Heart palpitations
- Hot flashes

- Chronic indigestion
- Internal trembling
- Itching, crawling sensations on the skin
- Joint pain
- Muscular twitching or cramps
- Numbness
- Obesity
- Premenstrual symptoms
- Ringing in ears
- Sensitivity to light and noise
- Excessive sighing and yawning
- Difficulty sleeping
- Excessive sweating

How many of these symptoms do you have? (The resources in Chapter 17 direct you to Web sites that show a more complete listing of symptoms.) If you've experienced a few or more, congratulations: It proves that you're not the living dead. Everyone is bound to have some of these symptoms at some time. If you have a few, especially of short duration, don't worry. Even if you experience the symptoms fairly regularly, other conditions may be causing them. For instance, hot flashes may be due to the fact that you're a female of a certain age. And as for itching and crawling sensations on the skin — don't look now, but there's a spider on your arm. (Not everything under the sun can be blamed on low blood sugar.)

Some symptoms can indicate a serious problem. See a doctor immediately if you experience dizziness, numbness, fainting, or convulsions.

PMS? Yes!

Premenstrual syndrome (PMS) is often associated with increased appetite, a craving for sweets, headaches, fatigue, and heart palpitations — in fact, all the symptoms of hypoglycemia. It's no wonder. Glucose tolerance tests given to premenstrual subjects showed excess insulin in response to sugar consumption. It appears that women who suffer from PMS have incidents of hypoglycemia that correlate with their menstrual cycles. If you're a woman who has experienced PMS, you know that you often crave something sweet and simple, such as sugar and flour, just before your period. It's the low blood sugar talking. Most women who devour sugar and simple starches experience stress, anxiety, and moodiness just before their periods — 80 to 90 percent, according to some research. The problem is easily rectified by changing your diet. Try to follow the diet recommended for hypoglycemics (see Chapter 6), especially when you feel an attack of PMS coming on.

Strange, You Don't Look Deranged: Emotional Symptoms

A woman placed an emergency call to her doctor in the middle of the night. She was generally a very well-mannered woman — except you wouldn't know it to listen to her then. She was in hysterics about her husband's infidelities. The next day she arrived at the clinic and, evidently distraught, stripped off all her clothes. As it turns out, she was a diabetic who had inadvertently taken too much insulin. She had a severe hypoglycemic reaction.

Most cases are not so dramatic (though diabetic hypoglycemia is generally much more serious than chronic cases of hypoglycemia). Nevertheless, people do behave in a bizarre manner when their tanks are running on empty (or when their blood glucose is low). You can't run without fuel and you accept that. So how can you expect your brain to work without the proper fuel — and in the case of that hefty gray matter (described further in Chapter 2), the fuel of choice is glucose. Starve your poor brain and you may have bizarre behavioral symptoms that can look like dementia, paranoia, or even schizophrenia.

Here's an extensive (but by no means complete) list of mental symptoms that can be induced by hypoglycemia:

- Antisocial behavior
- Circular thinking
- Constant worrying
- Difficulty in concentration
- Emotional fragility
- Exhaustion
- Feeling on edge
- Feelings of going mad or insane
- Feelings of inadequacy
- Forgetfulness
- Indecisiveness
- Irritability

- Lack of sex drive
- Low tolerance for stress
- Mental confusion
- Moodiness
- Negative thoughts and attitudes
- Nervousness
- Night terrors, nightmares
- Phobias
- Restlessness
- Suicidal thoughts or tendencies
- Temper tantrums

Of course, everyone experiences some of these emotional states at some time or other. (If you're convinced that you don't, ask your loved ones: They'll tell you otherwise!) What you should look out for is regular and extended bouts with these symptoms. By following the dietary guidelines and keeping a food journal like the one discussed in Chapter 6, you can make correlations to the foods, moods, and behaviors that affect you.

Seek professional help immediately if you experience suicidal thoughts/tendencies and mental confusion.

Unmasking Hypoglycemia's Hidden Faces

It may seem as though hypoglycemia is blamed for just about every condition under the sun. Maybe the stock market dive will eventually be attributed to low blood sugar. (The idea isn't as far-fetched as you may think. During the "bubble economy," some people speculated that the sky-rocketing economy was caused in part by investors feeling terribly optimistic after taking Prozac.)

What's confounding about hypoglycemia is that practically every one of its symptoms can be caused by other *pathological conditions* — namely, diseases and illnesses that have other causes. If you're suffering from symptoms that are suggestive of hypoglycemia, one of the following may be true:

- ✔ Hypoglycemia may be the hidden cause. In other words, you have these symptoms because you have hypoglycemia.

- ✔ The "hypoglycemic symptom" may indicate a different illness. The symptoms you have are the result of a different condition, not hypoglycemia.

- ✔ Hypoglycemia is paired with another condition. You have two conditions, one of which is hypoglycemia. In these cases, hypoglycemia may lead to the other condition, or the other condition may lead to hypoglycemia.

Untangling what's caused by what can be quite tricky, because the symptoms can overlap. For example, persistent fatigue, mood disorders, and brain dysfunctions, such as impaired memory and concentration — all hallmarks of hypoglycemia — are also symptoms of hypothyroidism and chronic fatigue syndrome. We can't cover every single condition related to hypoglycemia, so the following sections discuss a few of the major ones.

If you see little or no improvement in your condition after several months of following a hypoglycemic diet (see Chapter 6), you should suspect one or more of the other syndromes we discuss in the following sections. You don't have to worry about harming yourself if you stick to a hypoglycemic diet. It's a safe and sound way of eating. Unlike fad diets, the hypoglycemic diet can only improve your health, not hurt it.

Food reactions

If your doctor mentions food reactions, she's not talking about your food likes and dislikes. She's referring to allergies and a physical intolerance to certain foods. When you're allergic to a food, eating it provokes a reaction, such as an outbreak of rashes.

Even if you're not truly allergic to a substance, your body may still react to it. For instance, if you've ever eaten at a Chinese restaurant and hours later experienced headaches, nausea, dizziness, and other uncomfortable symptoms, it could be a reaction to MSG (monosodium glutamate), which is used for seasoning in many Chinese dishes.

Overlapping syndromes: Fibromyalgia, candidasis, and chronic fatigue

Teasing out the different symptoms is rather like trying to untangle a ball of yarn. A lot of syndromes overlap. This is particularly true of fibromyalgia, candidasis, and chronic fatigue syndrome, which share so many symptoms.

Fibromyalgia

Fibromyalgia syndrome (FMS) is a disorder that affects mostly women. The cause is still unknown. Patients typically suffer from fatigue, irritability, nervousness, depression, anxiety, sleep disorder, and cognitive and memory impairment. Many fibromyalgia patients also have a blood sugar imbalance.

How can you tell FMS from hypoglycemia? Through your pain (which former President Clinton could feel, or so he said). Although hypoglycemia can cause some muscle ache and joint pain, FMS patients generally ache all over: They experience pain in the muscles, ligaments, and tendons. They have spots on the body (called *tender points*) that — ouch! — hurt when pressed with enough pressure to whiten the thumbnail. They may also have genitourinary (cystitis, vaginal spasms, and so on) and gastrointestinal complaints (bloating, gas, constipation alternating with diarrhea). Interested in knowing more? Check out *Fibromyalgia For Dummies,* by Roland Staud, MD, and Christine Adamec (Wiley Publishing).

Candidasis

Your immune system and the presence of beneficial bacteria in your gut usually inhibit the overgrowth of *candida,* a fungi normally found in the body, particularly in the mouth, vagina, and intestinal tract.

If you're stressed, have an infection, experience a nutritional imbalance, or regularly use birth control pills, cortisone, or antibiotics over a long period of time, candida can proliferate and change to a fungoid form. Some people believe that this fungoid form can damage the intestinal lining and produce a wide range of symptoms (many of which are the same as the symptoms caused by hypoglycemia).

It should be noted, however, that nothing proves that candidasis exists as a disease state, and many doctors, including Dr. Chow (this book's co-author) are extremely careful about making a diagnosis of candidasis. Be wary of practitioners who readily blame candida for all kinds of health problems. Take a careful medical history and keep a meticulously accurate food journal. (See Chapter 6 for information on how to keep your own food journal.)

You may have reason to suspect candida if you have a few of the following conditions:

- ✔ Recurrent yeast infections
- ✔ Vaginal burning, itching, or discharge that proves resistant to treatment
- ✔ History of cortisone or antibiotic therapy
- ✔ History of thrush or chronic cystitis
- ✔ Symptoms of hypoglycemia that prove resistant to treatment

Going on a hypoglycemic diet can be very helpful if you think that you have candidasis. In addition, you should also avoid foods that contain yeast or are made with a fermentation process, including mature cheeses, vinegar, mushrooms, yogurt, sauerkraut, soy sauce, honey, oranges, and pickles.

Chronic fatigue syndrome

To make matters even more complex, *chronic fatigue syndrome* (CFS) can coexist with fibromyalgia (and hypoglycemia can coexist quite merrily with both these syndromes). Some experts believe that FMS and CFS are actually the same.

A key CFS symptom is severe, unexplained fatigue that's not relieved by rest and that lasts for at least six or more consecutive months. Other symptoms may include cognitive problems (lack of concentration, memory loss), sore throat without signs of infection, unrestful sleep, muscle pain, and headaches.

Haggling with hypothyroidism

Are you overweight? Are you tired, irritable, and constipated? Do you have headaches or a bad case of premenstrual syndrome? Do you seem to be allergic to everything, and, for crying out loud, are you losing your hair?

If you are experiencing these symptoms, you may very well have *hypothyroidism,* a condition where your thyroid gland doesn't produce enough of the hormone that regulates your metabolism. When you have too little thyroid hormone, you may experience depression, chronic fatigue, circulatory problems, compulsive overeating, and irritable bowel syndrome (whose symptoms include gas with alternating constipation and diarrhea).

 According to some practitioners, hypothyroidism is eight times more common in women than in men, and — listen up now — it's also an associated condition of hypoglycemia. In other words, low blood sugar can be caused by hypothyroidism, in which case you need to get it taken care of as soon as possible. You should change your diet, as well. It's always a good idea to eat wholesome, nourishing foods.

 The expected signs and symptoms of hypothyroidism aren't always present. The only way you can really be sure that you have the condition is to have some tests done. The free thyroxine (FT4) and the thyroid-stimulating hormone (TSH) tests are the most accurate and sensitive tests for determining thyroid function. In addition, ask your doctor to administer a TRH stimulation test. It's much more sensitive to thyroid hormone deficiencies than are standard measures, which only show very serious health conditions.

If your thyroid is indeed functioning below par, it can lead to hypoglycemia. As you know, hypoglycemia creates major imbalances in the body. When your hormones are off kilter, your body tries to compensate. The adrenal glands work extra to make up for the sluggish metabolism and the blood sugar imbalances. Before long, they get worn out. If they do wear out, you may develop a third condition: hypoadrenalism.

Joining the hypo bandwagon: Hypoadrenalism

Hypoadrenalism (hypoadrenia), or adrenal insufficiency, occurs when your adrenal glands become depleted, causing a decrease in the output of adrenal hormones. The extreme form of this condition, known as *Addison's disease,* can be life threatening if untreated. Fortunately it's quite rare, but if you do have it, you're in good company. President John Kennedy had adrenal insufficiency most of his life.

Less severe forms of low adrenal function (also called *adrenal fatigue*) can cause weight gain, fatigue, sleep disturbances, and panic attacks. And yes, these symptoms do sound disturbingly similar to the hypoglycemic symptoms. Modern medicine (mainstream Western medical practice) doesn't recognize the low-end, non-Addison's adrenal fatigue as a distinct syndrome. But many healthcare practitioners claim to have seen many patients who suffer from diminished activity of the adrenal glands. And — here's the link to hypoglycemia — they believe that sluggish adrenal function can lead to low blood sugar.

In most cases, following the recommended dietary and lifestyle changes described in this book can help with adrenal fatigue. If it doesn't, go to a nutritionally oriented medical doctor or naturopath. (Chapter 4 deals with lab tests, and Chapter 5 talks about alternative health practitioners.)

Hypoglycemia and Diabetes — Flip Sides of the Same Coin?

If you remember one thing from this book, make sure it's this: Insulin plays a critical role in your metabolism, which is directly related to your health, energy, and well-being. Hormones such as insulin, even a tiny amount, have incredibly powerful effects on the body.

Both diabetics and hypoglycemics have a glitch in their insulin functioning. Because insulin sweeps away blood sugar, excess insulin can lead to a drop in blood sugar. Sugars and simple starches trigger a greater insulin response than other foods, which is one reason why hypoglycemics are advised to stay away from them.

Syndrome flowchart

Although it's still a point of discussion, many researchers believe that hypoglycemia can be seen as a pre-diabetic form of glucose intolerance, which can eventually develop into full-blown diabetes in people who are genetically predisposed to diabetes. In other words, diabetes and hypoglycemia may fall on the continuum of the same degenerative disease (see Figure 3-1).

It starts with impaired glucose tolerance and then develops into insulin resistance. People with insulin resistance often also suffer from heart risk factors such as elevated blood pressure, low HDL cholesterol (the "good" kind), and abdominal obesity. Some researchers have begun calling a collection of these features *Syndrome X.* Bear in mind that there's no clear-cut point where one syndrome ends and the next one begins.

- ✔ **Impaired glucose tolerance.** This is a pre-diabetic condition in which the body is no longer able to use glucose well. The cells are beginning to lose their sensitivity to insulin, and they don't readily respond when insulin tries to deliver glucose to them, so the body produces more insulin.

- ✔ **Insulin resistance.** Even as the body is producing more insulin, the cells are losing their sensitivity to insulin. It's the task of insulin to deliver blood sugar to cells, but blood sugar remains in the bloodstream even when the cells stop responding.

- ✔ **Syndrome X.** Sounds like a mystery novel, doesn't it? Although you're not dealing with a murder mystery here, Syndrome X can indeed be deadly. This pre-diabetic condition is also known as *insulin resistance syndrome* or *metabolic cardiovascular risk syndrome* (MCVS). The underlying problem in people with Syndrome X is that their body is insensitive to insulin. (Think of it as insulin resistance with a few other "baddies" thrown in.) Other characteristics of Syndrome X include elevated blood cholesterol and *triglycerides* (fatty acids that normally circulate in the blood) and high blood pressure.

- ✔ **Diabetes (type 2).** This condition is a chronic syndrome of impaired fat, carbohydrate, and protein metabolism due to insufficient secretion of insulin or to insulin resistance. Blood sugar level remains elevated after fasting.

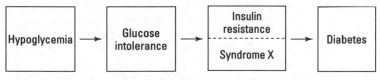

Figure 3-1: The possible progression of syndromes.

Types of diabetes

Some researchers suspect that 60 percent of people who suffer from hypoglycemia become diabetics. The two main types of diabetes are

- ✔ **Type 1.** This autoimmune disease develops when the pancreas stops producing insulin. It may also be caused by a viral infection.

✔ **Type 2.** This type of diabetes and hypoglycemia are like mirror images of each other. You may think of diabetes and hyoglycemia as part of the continuum of a progressive disease, with hypoglycemia at one end and diabetes at the other. Many practitioners believe that hypoglycemia can develop into type 2 diabetes, although this is a matter of debate. However, because obesity is a major contributing factor to type 2 diabetes, switching to a healthy diet can reduce your risk factor.

If you have a brother or sister with type 2 diabetes, you have about a 40 percent chance of getting the illness. If you have one parent with the disease, you have a 10 percent chance of getting it. While genetic inheritance causes type 2 diabetes, diet and lifestyle can help prevent it. Excess weight and lack of exercise can trigger diabetes, so pay attention to your diet and work out regularly.

If you're a low blood sugar sufferer, check into your family's medical history. When you look at the family medical history of hypoglycemics, you often find that they have close family members with either hypoglycemia or type 2 diabetes. If you want to know more about diabetes, check out *Diabetes For Dummies,* by Alan L. Rubin, MD (Wiley). The book gives a thorough explanation of type 1 and type 2 diabetes.

Snacking before bed: It's a go

Insulin regulation plays a role in your sleeping habits. If you're prone to low blood sugar, you may often have nightmares, night sweats, and sleeplessness. When you go without eating for many hours during nighttime, your blood glucose can plunge. This plunge in blood glucose levels drop kicks your adrenals into gear. Your adrenals then release adrenaline as a secondary energy source. Because adrenaline is a stimulatory hormone, it keeps you from having a sound, peaceful sleep. To avoid the effects of adrenaline, have a light snack just before going to bed. Yogurt or cottage cheese are good choices. If you have a weight problem, make sure that the snack isn't something that's high in calories. Remember, you don't need to eat a lot — and avoid foods, such as simple starches, that will cause your body to produce too much insulin.

Part II
Getting a Diagnosis: Do I or Don't I?

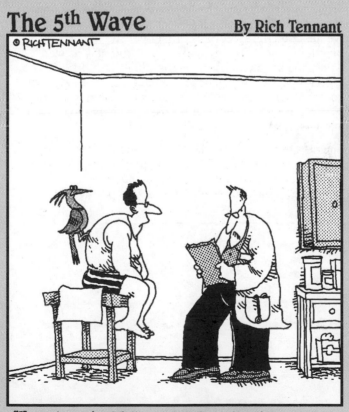

The 5th Wave · By Rich Tennant

© RICHTENNANT

"Hypoglycemia? Well, maybe. But, like that pain in your shoulder, it could be a lot of things."

In this part . . .

Perhaps it was a chance remark or something you read; you have some cause to suspect that you or your loved one may be hypoglycemic. This section can help you determine if you suffer from this condition. We describe the symptoms and cover the underlying biochemistry behind hypoglycemia. You may as well have a nodding acquaintance with the different types of hypoglycemia, so we briefly describe each one. We help you sort through all the complexities and permutations of this syndrome and rule out other possible causes for what's ailing you.

Because hypoglycemia means low blood sugar, we talk about sugar a lot: what it is, how your body metabolizes it, and what it does to your health. Ah, such a sweet subject, sugar. But it's a bittersweet one, as this part tells you.

Chapter 4

Getting the Lowdown on Low Blood Sugar

● ●

In This Chapter
▶ Diagnosing low blood sugar
▶ Trying the trial diet
▶ Figuring out what glucose tolerance tests can do
▶ Detecting food reactions

● ●

*P*erhaps you've been suffering from vague symptoms, like those described in Chapter 3, that you think may indicate hypoglycemia. Maybe you suspect that your body can't metabolize carbohydrates properly. Or, maybe you're just the curious type. This chapter may provide a moment of truth: Here you find tools that help determine whether you have hypoglycemia. Following the guidelines in this chapter can help you make as good an assessment of your symptoms. (Of course, see your doctor for the best assessment.)

You see, diagnosing hypoglycemia isn't as definitive as diagnosing diabetes. There's no absolute standard for determining hypo- glycemia. You can take the glucose tolerance test (GTT), but it's not an infallible tool. Your doctor should also review your medical history and symptoms. In that sense, it's very much like other con- troversial diagnoses, such as chronic fatigue syndrome and fibromyalgia. (In fact, those syndromes may often be associated with low blood sugar. If you want to know more, see Chapter 3.)

Taking the tests in this chapter does not substitute for seeing a doctor. Even if you test negatively here, see a doctor if you suspect that you have hypoglycemia or any other disorder.

Poking and Prodding Yourself

Before you go gallivanting off to your doctor, you can take a questionnaire in the comfort and privacy of your own home. In addition to the questionnaire, you may want to consider going on the trial diet, which can give you even more information about the state of your health, making it easier for your doctor to arrive at a diagnosis.

Filling in the circles: A questionnaire

Before you fill out the questionnaire, make a photocopy of it, or leave yourself enough room to write down answers at a later date. Make sure that you write down the date you're taking the test; you should take the test every three weeks to keep track of your progress. All right, now you're primed and prepped for the following questionnaire.

Answer Yes or No to the following questions:

Date:	Yes	No
Do you often crave sweets?		
Do you generally feel ravenously hungry between meals?		
Do you worry constantly or experience unprovoked anxieties?		
Do you have trouble sleeping?		
Are you irritable if you miss a meal?		
Do you feel tired, weak, or shaky if you miss a meal?		
Do you feel tired an hour or so after eating?		
Do you get dizzy when you stand suddenly?		
Do you experience vertigo (dizziness)?		
Do you usually feel fatigued or exhausted?		
Do you experience internal trembling?		
Are you often confused?		
Do you have heart palpitations?		
Do you get frequent headaches?		

	Yes	No
Are you often forgetful?		
Do you have frequent crying spells?		
Do you have difficulty concentrating?		
Do you experience blurred vision?		
Do you have depression or mood swings?		
Do you feel as though you're going crazy?		
Do you have frequent backaches?		
Do you often have problems with digestion?		
Are you apt to engage in asocial or antisocial behavior?		
Are you indecisive?		
Do you get frequent leg cramps?		
Do you often experience muscle pains or muscular twitching?		
Do you often feel lightheaded?		
Do you experience numbness?		
Do you usually have cold hands and/or feet?		
Do you have fainting spells or blackouts?		
Do you have convulsions?		
Do you experience bloating?		
Are you overweight? (See the "Figuring out your BMI" sidebar to calculate.)		

Scoring: Add 1 for each Yes answer.

<5: Probably not hypoglycemic.

6 to 19: Hypoglycemia is likely.

>20: Hypoglycemia is extremely likely.

This test is a general guideline. In addition, if you have diabetics or hypoglycemics in your family, you're probably prone to blood sugar imbalance and other manifestations of hypoglycemia. Even if you have only a few severe or recurrent symptoms, you may be hypoglycemic. An excellent way to find out if you are hypoglycemic is to try this chapter's diet and see whether your symptoms (see Chapter 3) diminish or clear up. Following the diet will give your doctor more information to work with.

See a doctor immediately if you have symptoms such as vertigo, blurred vision, numbness, blackouts, palpitations, or convulsions. These symptoms can indicate another, more urgent, health matter.

Eating by trial

Trying out the following diet for at least 20 days can give you a fairly good indication of the likelihood of hypoglycemia.

- ✔ Avoid all sugars, stimulants, and heavy starch foods — this includes pasta, bread, corn, rice, and potatoes. (Be sure to read labels on everything, because prepared foods often contain hidden sugar.)

- ✔ Don't eat deep fried foods, breading, or sauces, and stay away from all desserts and fruits.

- ✔ Don't drink alcoholic beverages.

- ✔ If you smoke, try to at least cut back.

- ✔ You can eat as many vegetables as you like.

This diet is just a test to help you find out whether the seemingly unrelated symptoms you have are due to hypoglycemia, which is basically an underlying *metabolic disorder* that makes your body incapable of handling carbohydrates properly. (See Chapters 1 and 2 for more about what hypoglycemia is.) This diet isn't the prescribed diet for hypoglycemia (although similarities exist), and you don't have to stay on it forever. You may experience a temporary worsening of your symptoms in the first week or so, but they should ease up eventually.

Fill out the questionnaire (earlier in this chapter) again at the end of the diet's trial period. If you have fewer symptoms, or if your symptoms become less intense or disappear, it's a good indication that you have hypoglycemia, particularly if you've already had all kinds of medical tests and nothing was found to be wrong. (If that's the case, you may want to check out the information about doctors in Chapter 5.)

As with any task worth doing, going on the trial diet may be challenging, but you can make it easier by exercising (see Chapter 8), using meditation and deep breathing techniques (see Chapter 9), and following Chapter 16's helpful hints for making life more manageable. In fact, you may be pleasantly surprised by how much better you feel and how much more energy you have.

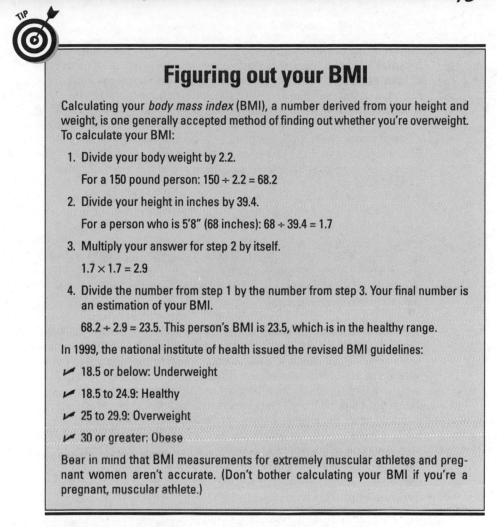

Figuring out your BMI

Calculating your *body mass index* (BMI), a number derived from your height and weight, is one generally accepted method of finding out whether you're overweight. To calculate your BMI:

1. Divide your body weight by 2.2.

   For a 150 pound person: 150 ÷ 2.2 = 68.2

2. Divide your height in inches by 39.4.

   For a person who is 5'8" (68 inches): 68 ÷ 39.4 = 1.7

3. Multiply your answer for step 2 by itself.

   1.7 × 1.7 = 2.9

4. Divide the number from step 1 by the number from step 3. Your final number is an estimation of your BMI.

   68.2 ÷ 2.9 = 23.5. This person's BMI is 23.5, which is in the healthy range.

In 1999, the national institute of health issued the revised BMI guidelines:

✔ 18.5 or below: Underweight

✔ 18.5 to 24.9: Healthy

✔ 25 to 29.9: Overweight

✔ 30 or greater: Obese

Bear in mind that BMI measurements for extremely muscular athletes and pregnant women aren't accurate. (Don't bother calculating your BMI if you're a pregnant, muscular athlete.)

Getting the 411 on the Glucose Tolerance Tests

Despite their drawbacks, lab tests can be used as part of the diagnostic procedure. Two tests can help diagnose hypoglycemia: the glucose tolerance test (GTT) and glucose insulin tolerance test (G-ITT). Keep in mind, though, that neither test is considered conclusive.

The G-ITT is a standard GTT coupled with the measurement of insulin levels; it's much more sensitive in spotting faulty sugar metabolism. Studies show that people with suspected diabetes or hypoglycemia who test normal when only the GTT is taken will show up as abnormal on the G-ITT.

The GTT can diagnose both diabetes and hypoglycemia, although it's rarely used to test for diabetes. These days, GTT isn't even considered the instrument of choice for diagnosing hypoglycemia. Because of the controversy over the criteria for evaluating the GTT, no lab tests can conclusively diagnose hypoglycemia. Looking only at the blood sugar values can give skewed results. It can flag healthy people as hypoglycemics; conversely, hypoglycemics may be erroneously told they're healthy. Some people have hypo symptoms even though their lowest numbers are in the normal range.

The glucose tolerance tests are usually conducted in the morning, after you've *fasted* (gone without food) for 10 to 12 hours. A blood sample is taken so that doctors can see what your blood sugar level is on an empty stomach. Next, you're asked to drink a solution of about 75 grams of glucose (sugar) in 300 ml (milliliters) of water. After an hour (sometimes half an hour), a blood sample is drawn again. Blood samples are then taken again every hour for the next three to six hours.

The most important aspects of the GTT are the symptoms that occur during the test and, to some extent, the relief of these symptoms after eating. Both of these factors need to be taken into consideration along with the blood glucose levels measured during the test. The fact is, some people may have hypoglycemic symptoms even though their blood sugar level falls comfortably within the normal range. An individual may go totally nuts and yet have a virtually identical glucose tolerance test reading to someone who is calm and collected. Results that are considered normal may not necessarily be normal for you. Your body may not be able to function properly with a blood sugar level that is considered normal by medical doctors.

The GTT is no picnic in the park. (Ditto for the G-ITT!) It's long, it's stressful, and for those of you who have a severe case of hypoglycemia, your symptoms will probably flare up during the test. If you want to spare yourself the time and expense of taking the tests, just try out the two-week trial diet in Chapter 6. Many hypoglycemia veterans attest that how you feel while you're on the diet gives you at least as good a clue — or even better — to whether you're hypoglycemic than do the tests.

To make an accurate assessment of either the GTT or the G-ITT, it is important for your doctor to observe how fast your blood sugar drops (rather than how low it drops). Basically, hypoglycemia is suspected if the natural rise is followed by a rapid drop below the normal fasting range. The lower and faster it drops, the more severe the condition. A person may experience more problems if his sugar level drops from 200 milligrams (mg) to 100 mg in one hour or less, than if it drops from 100 mg to 45 mg in two or three hours.

The advantages to taking either the GTT or the G-ITT, should the results indicate that you have an abnormality, are

- If you need to convince your employer or your family and friends that your hypoglycemia is not all in your head, you'll have medical documentation for proving your case. (See Chapter 12 for more about work.)

- It's likely to motivate you to make the necessary dietary changes.

- You can use the results to predict when your blood sugar will dip, and then you can schedule your snacks accordingly.

- The test can indicate whether further testing is needed to determine if there's a serious organic cause for your hypo-glycemia, such as a tumor of the pancreas. Chances are that you don't have cancer of the pancreas, because it's a rare con-dition, but it's always a good idea to rule out other causes. Better safe than sorry, as they say.

Types of Hypo

The rise and fall of the sugar level in the bloodstream indicates what type of hypoglycemia you have.

Organic

With this type of hypoglycemia, your blood sugar level when you have been fasting is invariably low. (The *fasting level* is the amount of sugar in the your blood when a sample of blood is drawn after *fasting* — not eating anything — for 10 to 12 hours, and before you're given the glucose solution to drink.) The symptoms are usu-ally continuous.

G-ITT this test

In addition to testing your glucose level, we strongly recommend that you have your insulin or epinephrine level measured at the same time (via the G-ITT), because hypoglycemic symptoms often correlate better with elevations of these hormones than with blood sugar levels. People with hypoglycemia often have food sensitivi-ties that can contribute to their symptoms. The tests for food reactions are described in the sidebar, "Being a Little Food Sensitive," later in this chapter.

This type of hypoglycemia warrants further investigation to determine whether the you have an enlarged pancreas, tumors of the pancreas, or possibly other causes that are unrelated to what you do or do not eat.

Reactive

With this type of hypoglycemia, symptoms fluctuate according to the food you eat, the time of day when you eat, and so on. In reactive hypoglycemia, the level of sugar in your blood when you have been fasting — before drinking the liquid glucose — may be normal or even a little above what's considered normal. Your body then overreacts to the glucose by producing too much insulin, which causes the fall in blood sugar. (That's why it's called *reactive.*)

Relative

Relative hypoglycemia is a condition where your blood sugar is low in relation to your fasting level. The group of people most often misdiagnosed as normal suffer from relative hypoglycemia. For example, you are said to have relative hypoglycemia if

- ✔ Your blood sugar falls 20 mg or more below your fasting level and you experience symptoms.
- ✔ Your blood sugar falls 50 mg or more within one hour and you experience symptoms.
- ✔ Your blood sugar increases by 20 mg or less after ingesting the glucose and then falls to at least 20 mg below your fasting level.

Testing, Testing

No lab tests can conclusively diagnose hypoglycemia. That's because of the controversy over the criteria for evaluating the test. Looking only at blood sugar values can give skewed results, flagging healthy people as hypoglycemics; and conversely, hypoglycemics may be told they're healthy. Some people will have hypo symptoms even with their lowest numbers in the normal range.

Despite the drawbacks, lab tests like the GTT and G-ITTcan be part of the diagnosing. Neither of these tests is conclusive.

Before you take either the GTT or the G-ITT, find out if your insurance will pick up the cost. Most insurance policies cover GTTs for diabetics; they may also reimburse you if your doctor confirms a diagnosis of hypoglycemia. But unless you're enrolled under a generous policy, chances are that you'll have to pay out-of-pocket.

Pre-test

You're going to take the GTT or the G-ITT and see what's going on with your body.

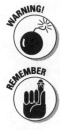

Ask a friend or family member to take you to the clinic and pick you up after the test. Because you may have severe reactions to the test, it can be dangerous for you to drive home or take public transportation.

Keep these things in mind:

✔ Tell your doctor about any prescription medications you're currently taking, especially diuretic drugs, anti-epileptic drugs, contraceptives, and drugs containing cortisone or aspirin.

✔ Arrange to have extra blood samples taken while you're having obvious symptoms, such as rapid pulse, sweating, or sudden weakness, at least 15 minutes before the next blood sample is to be drawn. When you get these symptoms, call a nurse immediately.

✔ Arrange to get a personal copy of your results.

✔ Make sure that you get the six-hour test and not the shorter three-, four-, or even five-hour test. For some individuals, blood sugar may not fall below the normal level until after the fourth or fifth hour. Yes, this means that the test will be an all-day affair. Here's what you should prepare:

  • Good reading materials (for helping pass the time)

  • Food to eat when the test is over (to help level out your blood sugar)

  • A notebook or some papers (to help pass the time; also good for adding to your food journal later)

  • A pen (because trying to write with crayons is tough)

  • A watch (so you can record your body's rhythms and see the light at the end of the testing tunnel)

You can't touch any food until the test is over. If you do, the results will be invalidated. You can drink only water.

Mid-test

So you have on your comfy clothes, you're clutching a new book, and your tummy is rumbling. Here's what to expect when you show up at the clinic:

1. **Blood is drawn to take a *baseline blood sugar measurement* (the amount of sugar in your bloodstream after an overnight fast).**

   The doctor needs to have baseline measurement in order to find out what your body does with the sugar. If the thought of needles freaks you out, refer to Chapter 10 and practice some of the stress-relieving exercises.

2. **You're given a glucose solution to drink.**

   It's presented in a bottle containing about 75 grams of glucose (sugar) in 300 ml (milliliters) of water. You don't have to drink it in one gulp, but you want to swallow it reasonably quickly; don't nurse it like a cup of latte. You'll only be asked to drink this one bottle.

   Don't lie down during the test unless you're very weak. Blood sugar tends to remain high if you don't move at all, so lying down may skew the results. If possible, walk around the clinic and stretch out your legs. Just make sure that you get back in time for the drawing of blood.

3. **Blood is drawn again at 30 minutes and at 1 hour, and then hourly for up to 6 hours.**

   The blood samples are examined for their actual sugar content at specific intervals. The samples show how your body utilizes sugar.

4. **You're informed when the test is over.**

5. **You're told the results after your doctor gets them from the lab.**

Post-test

You're done. Take a breath. You'll probably be tired after the test, so don't schedule anything demanding that night. You may want to skip your kickboxing class. Of course, if you're feeling bright and chipper and raring to go, don't hold back. Go challenge the neigh-borhood wrestling champ if you want. As long as it's legal, feel free to do whatever you like.

It's not common, but some patients experience vertigo, disorienta-tion, and other severe symptoms during the test. Some start crying uncontrollably, get into an argument with the nurse, or otherwise engage in bizarre behavior. If you experience any of these symp-toms, don't be alarmed.

Write down any symptoms or adverse effects that you experience during the test, such as dizziness, abdominal cramps, irritability, depression and so on, and the time that they occurred. Keeping track of this information is crucial, as it will aid in interpreting your test results. You'll be able to compare the reactions that you expe-rienced during the test to your blood sugar levels at the time of the reactions. This is a good reason to have someone there with you: Your companion can note such incidences, even if you're too far gone to write anything down.

Interpreting the results

To interpret the test, you need to understand how doctors meas-ure the amount of sugar in the blood.

Results are shown per 100 milliliters (ml) of blood. Here are the spans for fasting blood sugar levels:

- 80–110 mg: The normal span.
- 110–125 mg: Impaired glucose tolerance.
- >126 mg: Raises the suspicion of diabetes.

More blood? Sure, we'll take it

You can ask for blood to be drawn every half hour to increase the accuracy of the test, but the test will cost more — and you'll have many more lovely puncture wounds on your arms. Something to consider: Instead of having your blood tested every half hour, make a special request to have a specimen taken after 3½ hours. (It's not normally done, so you have to ask.) This specimen can reveal abnormalities that may be missed otherwise.

After you swallow the glucose drink, you're no longer considered to be fasting. The blood sugar level rises slightly in the healthy individual, perhaps to 120 mg, depending on where the fasting level was, and then falls back to the fasting level. For a short period of time, the blood sugar level drops slightly below the level it was at during fasting, and then it returns to normal fairly quickly.

The nonfasting blood sugar levels are recorded after 30 minutes and then every hour after you drink the glucose beverage:

- ✔ <140 mg: Normal.

- ✔ 140–199 mg: Impaired glucose tolerance.

- ✔ >200 mg: Indicates diabetes.

In the diabetic person, blood sugar comes down very slowly, returning to the fasting level after six or more hours. And what about hypoglycemics? Unfortunately, the criteria for diagnosing hypoglycemia is not so clear. Doctors can't agree on a specific number. However, right now hypoglycemia is officially recognized in an individual only if fasting blood sugar falls below 45 mg during a 72-hour fast.

Because hypoglycemics have so many different sugar curves, you should select a doctor who is specifically trained to treat hypoglycemia. (Chapter 5 has information on selecting the right doctor.) To make an accurate assessment of your health condition, it is important for your doctor to observe how fast the blood sugar drops rather than how low it drops.

Basically, if the natural rise of the blood sugar is followed by a rapid drop below the normal fasting range, hypoglycemia is suspected. The lower and the faster the blood sugar level drops, the more severe the condition. A person may experience more problems if the level drops from 200 mg to 100 mg in one hour or less, than if it drops from 100 mg to 45 mg in 2 or 3 hours. Some other factors to consider when diagnosing hypoglycemia are

- ✔ How fast does the blood sugar level return to normal?

- ✔ How long does the sugar level remain at the low point?

For instance, the blood sugar level may drop to a low 45, but if it recovers quickly and returns to the fasting level in about an hour, you may not even notice it, or you may experience only mild symptoms. You may have more severe symptoms if, say, your blood sugar drops to 65 mg and remains there for a few hours because it takes a long time to return to your fasting level.

Figure 4-1 shows what a hypoglycemic's curves may look like.

✔ Line A shows that the glucose level has fallen below 50 mg.

✔ Line B indicates that the level has fallen below the original fasting level of 80 mg.

✔ Line C shows a severe percentage drop in the short term.

✔ Line D stays below the fasting level of 100 mg for an extended time.

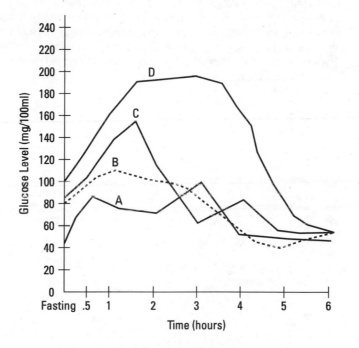

The following are considered hypoglycemic curves:

A: Glucose level falls below 50mg/dl.

B: Glucose level falls more than 30mg percent below fasting level

C: Glucose level shows severe percentage drop in short time.

D: Glucose level stays above fasting level for extended period.

Figure 4-1: Curves for hypoglycemia.

After you have a GTT test performed

1. **Ask your doctor to give you a copy of the results of your test.**

2. **Chart a graph.**

    You can see examples in Figures 4-1, 4-2, 4-3, 4-4, and 4-5.

3. **Compare the notes you took during the test to your blood sugar levels represented on the graph.**

4. **Go over the results with your doctor.**

One picture is worth a 1,000 words, so one graph should be good for at least 500. Figures 4-2 through 4-5 offer four sample graphs that give you an idea of what the tests look like. See just how sexy these glucose tolerance curves can be? You can tell how the rise and fall of the blood sugar level for diabetes, relative hypoglycemia, and flat glucose tolerance curves (considered a type of hypoglycemia) differ significantly from one another.

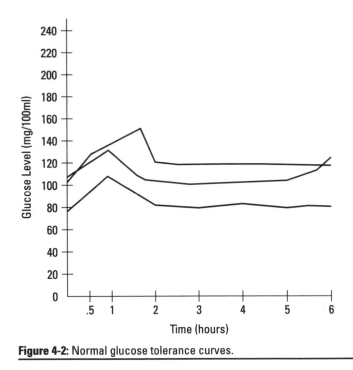

Figure 4-2: Normal glucose tolerance curves.

Don't pancreas

In some cases, patients show symptoms of having hypoglycemia that may be of organic origin. When you have hypoglycemia that is organic in origin, your glucose fasting level is invariably low. It's called *fasting hypoglycemia*, and it warrants further investigation to determine whether you have an enlarged pancreas or tumors of the pancreas. In contrast, the fasting level of glucose in a person with reactive hypoglycemia may be normal or even a little above normal. The body then overreacts to the glucose by producing too much insulin, which causes the fall in blood sugar.

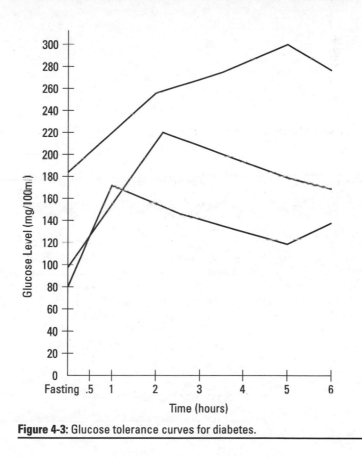

Figure 4-3: Glucose tolerance curves for diabetes.

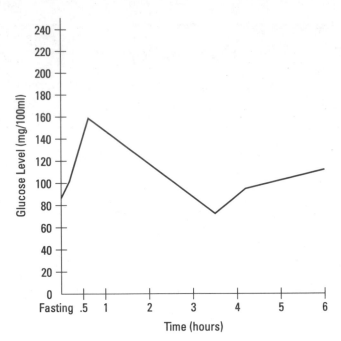

Figure 4-4: Relative hypoglycemia: The glucose level falls 50 mg or more below fasting levels in one hour.

Being a little food sensitive

If you want to be really thorough when getting tested for the cause of your hypoglycemia symptoms, consider getting tested for food reactions. Whether people can develop allergy-like reactions to common foods is still a matter of heated debate. So far, studies have failed to prove that food sensitivities can cause vague symptoms such as headaches, nasal congestgion, or fatigue. Most medical doctors scoff at the idea that people can suffer from delayed reactions to eating certain foods. Nonetheless, many practitioners familiar with hypoglycemia are convinced that food sensitivities can contribute to the symptoms.

Lab tests for food sensitivities can be quite expensive. And because there's so much disagreement about how valid they are, save your money: Use the elimination diet. It may clue you in on which foods are causing you problems.

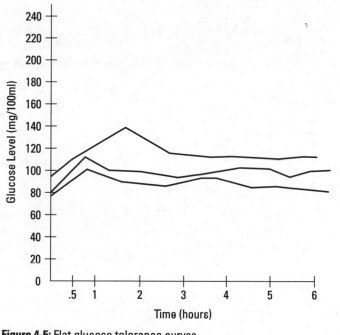

Figure 4-5: Flat glucose tolerance curves.

Chapter 5

Matching Up with the Right Doc

· ·

In This Chapter

▶ Finding the right doctor for you

▶ Deciding which specialist to see

▶ Preparing for doctor visits

▶ Considering alternative healing methods

· ·

All right. Unless you're highly unusual, you'd probably rather spend your day reclining seductively on a couch than you would trying to recline in a clinic waiting room. But hey, everyone has to do it sooner or later. Rather than jump to conclusions about your health, you owe it to yourself to get a thorough physical check-up to make sure that you get a proper diagnosis of your hypoglycemia symptoms. And you need to make sure that your low blood sugar isn't due to other *organic* causes (producing or involving alteration of an organ's structure) or something totally unrelated to hypoglycemia. Only when you've ruled out other illnesses can you begin the proper course of treatment. The danger of self-diagnosis is that you may be treating yourself for a problem that doesn't even exist, while the real disease goes untreated.

By the way, even if you're merely the friend or family member of someone with hypoglycemia, and you're feeling fine, if you haven't been to the doc for a check-up in a few years, we strongly recommend that you get one. (And no, we're not saying this because the co-author has a vested interest in hauling everyone's behind into a doctor's office.) Keeping on top of your health, with the help of your primary care physician (PCP), is extremely important. You can identify problems — and potential problems — earlier and nip them in the bud. Don't wait until you're in dire need of medical attention before you see a doctor; preventing problems is often easier than treating them.

Many people avoid the doctor's office because they're afraid of needles or of pain in general. We confess that *some* minor discomfort *may* be involved, depending on what tests your doctor administers, but standard physicals are pretty much pain free. And we promise you that the experience will be much less traumatic than that time you were abducted by space aliens. Honest. The medical staff is much more human, for one thing; they're basically nice folks who want you to feel comfortable and relaxed. (Most get into the profession because they want to help others; however, if the medical professional you visit makes Nurse Ratched from *One Flew Over the Cuckoo's Nest* seem like Florence Nightingale, you may want to switch to another clinic.)

Okay, okay — the lecture's over. Now go make an appointment with a doctor. Do you know who you should see? Maybe you're not sure. In that case, read on; this chapter helps you determine who you should hire (and maybe fire) and lets you know what to expect when you get a physical. If you'd rather see an alternative health practitioner, we have suggestions for finding one of those, too.

Hearing a Word from Our Sponsor

When dealing with your health, you have to be proactive and take charge. If you're too weak, fatigued, depressed, or whatever to muster up the energy and clarity of mind to orchestrate everything, assign someone you trust to take care of things for you. If no one in your family or circle of friends can do this, consider paying a professional, or perhaps a therapist or a life coach, to do it for you. Hiring a professional obviously costs extra money, but the expenses are only temporary. And you'll feel better — probably much sooner than you think.

After all is said and done, treating hypoglycemia is surprisingly simple and low-tech. Avoid refined sugars and starches, eat high-quality protein and whole, natural foods, and exercise regularly. Get a good belly laugh every day. Watch comedies. Read Dave Barry.

REMEMBER

Coming clean

Finding the healthcare provider of your dreams (hopefully not your nightmares!) is only the beginning. You're expected to tell your doctor everything connected to your health and follow her directions and advice.

If you've noticed any changes in your body, or you've made adjustments in your lifestyle or diet (good or bad), tell your doctor. If you have a drug habit or a drinking problem, you have to come clean. A doctor's office is no place for secrets. If you visit a doctor in the United States or other industrialized countries, whatever you tell a doctor will remain in her office, so don't worry about Aunt Thelma finding out about your deep, dark secrets. In less developed parts of the world such as China, you can't count on doctor/patient confidentiality. So you may want to first check out your legal rights.

Paging Dr. Perfection

You may have to put forth some effort when trying to find a good doctor for treating your symptoms of hypoglycemia. Aside from being competent and having the proper credentials, your doctor should be caring and compassionate.

You have several things to consider when choosing a doctor, not the least of which includes:

- Familiarity with hypoglycemia (or at least being open-minded about it)
- Belief in the importance of nutrition for maintaining good health
- Willingness to work with alternative healthcare practitioners
- Taking your health complaints seriously
- Spending the time to thoroughly evaluate your condition
- Listening carefully to what you say
- Encouraging you to ask questions
- Asking you effective questions
- Explaining things clearly and fully
- Anticipating your health problems
- Welcoming your participation in the treatment
- Flexibility (no, not the kind that lets him do the splits)

Add anything else that's truly important to you to this list. The location of the doctor's office, the hospital where the doctor treats patients, and the type of health insurance you have may all factor into your consideration. Avoid anyone who's dismissive of you and your concerns. Drop him or her back into the swamp for further evolution. You deserve better than that.

Now, how do you go about finding the right doc for you? Follow these steps:

1. **Ask around.**

   Ask friends, co-workers, relatives, or any other health professionals you know. Obviously, the people to ask are those individuals who have been treated for hypoglycemia. If you don't know anyone who has hypoglycemia, contact your local medical society, church, university medical centers, or other groups. (Chapter 17 gives some other great resources.)

   Get several names to choose from, just in case the doctor you select isn't currently taking new patients or doesn't participate in your health insurance plan.

2. **When someone recommends a doctor, ask that person specific questions.**

   - What is the doctor's area of expertise?

   - How would you describe the doctor's bedside manner?

   - What kind of experience did you have with the doctor?

3. **Set up an appointment just to talk with the doctor and ask questions.**

   Make sure you both understand that you're trying to decide on a doctor. You'll have to pay for the visit, but you may save yourself some money in the long run.

Unfortunately, many doctors think that the only hypoglycemia that's legitimate is the type of low blood sugar that's induced by diabetics who miscalculate the amount of insulin they need. If you're suffering from a chronic condition of hypoglycemia that can't be traced to an obvious cause, your doctor may be tempted to dismiss your complaints as being all in your mind. Should that happen, don't take it personally. Western medicine is used to treating illnesses aggressively with drugs and surgery rather than through diet and lifestyle modifications.

Let it roll off your back

If your doctor isn't sympathetic, don't take it personally. Understand where he or she is coming from. Some are trained to aggressively combat disease with drugs and surgery, not to look for nutritional or lifestyle factors. When patients come in with nonspecific complaints that are hard to pinpoint, some doctors may get very frustrated.

Here are some reasons why a doctor may not believe hypoglycemia is causing your symptoms:

✔ Hypoglycemia has been rampantly overdiagnosed.

✔ Experts disagree on exactly what constitutes hypoglycemia.

✔ Glucose tolerance tests (GTT) for hypoglycemia don't always show abnormally low levels of blood sugar.

✔ The array of symptoms are nonspecific (fatigue, dizziness, and depression, for example) and can have many different causes other than hypoglycemia.

✔ It's too easy for patients to ascribe everything on hypoglycemia, because it's associated with so many different symptoms.

✔ The symptoms associated with hypoglycemia can't be pinpointed to a specific dysfunction or damaged organs.

Choosing a Specialist, Any Specialist

So, have you confessed everything to your kind doctor? Are you wondering if you should see a specialist? Specialists offer many options.

Specialists have at least three years of specialty training, under supervision, after getting their MD (medical doctor) degree. Some specialists are primary care doctors, such as family physicians or *internists* (more on them in the next section). Other specialists concentrate on certain body systems, specific age groups, or complex scientific techniques.

A good way to find out about a doctor's expertise is to ask about her board certification. To be board certified after graduating from medical school, doctors have to pass an exam certifying them as specialists in certain fields of medicine. They also have to complete 150 hours of continuing medical education every three years and pass a comprehensive exam every seven years. (At least you know that they haven't forgotten everything they learned in med school.)

Family doctors and internists

What's the difference between an internist and a family physician?

- ✔ An *internist* is a doctor of adults who specializes in the diagnosis and treatment of nonsurgical ailments. You can find internists in hospitals and clinics. Some internists may specialize in other areas and become the friendly specialist that your illness calls for. These specialty areas may include arthritis, asthma, cancer, diabetes, and most surgical procedures.

- ✔ A *family physician* is basically a general practitioner (GP) who has done residency in family practice. Family physicians provide healthcare to individuals regardless of their age. They give you regular check-ups, and they diagnose and treat most patient problems. You can visit a family doctor for a glucose tolerance test, which is sometimes used to screen for hypoglycemia. (See Chapter 4 to find out more about glucose tolerance tests.) Family physicians can refer you to another specialist if they can't treat certain problems.

If you're not sure what you have, or you suspect that you have hypoglycemia, internists or family physicians are probably your best bet. Internists and physicians can schedule tests and refer you to hospitals and other specialists as needed. They'll discuss your treatment with your family (if appropriate) and anyone else involved in your healthcare. Their role is that of team leader.

Endocrinologists

Endocrinologists specialize in diseases and disorders of the endocrine system (hormones), which is involved in blood sugar regulation. Endocrinologists also treat diabetes, a condition that is connected to blood sugar regulation. Should you see an endocrinologist if you think that you have hypoglycemia?

Unless you have a glowing personal recommendation for an inno-vative endocrinologist with experience in hypoglycemia, an endocrinologist probably isn't your best bet. Why? Because, as specialists, endocrinologists are more familiar with serious ill-nesses and aren't usually attuned to identifying hypoglycemia's chronic conditions. If you want someone who is more attuned to hypoglycemia, you're better off with a general practitioner or a physician who focuses on diagnosing and treating the condition.

You may consider seeing an endocrinologist, though, if you're obese, and you fail to lose weight after following the hypoglycemic food program for several months. (Keep a food journal to make sure that you're not subconsciously cheating! Flip to Chapter 6 to see how to keep a journal.) You may be suffering from other metabolic or hor-monal imbalances. Endocrinologists are real pros at treating these conditions, as well as in identifying genetic or other factors (such as insulin resistance) that may be affecting your weight.

At any rate, you're probably better off going to a doctor who already has your medical history. Spend some time going over your symptoms and all your health concerns. Your doctor can direct you to the proper specialist should you need one.

Preparing Shows You're Caring (about Yourself)

So you've talked to your friends and decided on a potential doctor. Before making an appointment, call the office and find out about the doctor's fees, payment procedures, and insurance coverage. (Before you make an inference, read more about insurance in *Insurance For Dummies,* by Jack Hungelmann, from Wiley Publishing.)

In order to have the most productive visit possible, prepare the fol-lowing items before your first appointment:

✔ **A list of all your symptoms.** (Chapter 4 can help you in this arena.)

Don't just leave your list of symptoms on the kitchen table; bring it with you! Chronic hypoglycemia can make you a wee bit forgetful, and the list can help jog your memory. You can show the doctor the list, but flesh out your symptoms by describing as completely as possible the timing, frequency, intensity, and duration of your problems.

When relating your symptoms, go from the general to the specific. Describe the following:

- How it feels, followed by facts that you can see or touch, such as body temperature (You'll impress the heck out of the doc!)

- When you first started to notice the symptom

- The time of the day that it occurs

- Whether you see a pattern

- How the various symptoms are affecting your life and work

✔ **Your medical history (including dates for surgeries, hospitalizations, and major illnesses) and your family's medical history.**

Consult your family beforehand, so that you can construct as accurate and complete a medical history as possible. You may think that you know your family's medical history, but your parents or grandparents may have had illnesses that you weren't aware of. Grill your parents and siblings if you have to.

✔ **The names of medications you're taking.** (Give either the generic or brand name, but skip any pet names you call them.)

Your list should include any and all prescribed and *over-the-counter (OTC) meds* (medications you don't need a prescription for), vitamins, herbal supplements (see Chapter 8 for more on these treatments), and birth control. (Take samples of any herbs you're taking if you're unsure of the name. This is particularly true if you're also seeing a Chinese herbalist.)

✔ **A list of any treatments that you're receiving from other healthcare practitioners.**

These healthcare practitioners may include chiropractors, acupuncturists, dietitians, homeopaths, naturopaths, and osteopaths (but no psychopaths, please!).

✔ **A pen and paper for taking notes.**

Jot down the most important points that your doctor covers, including advice or recommendations. Forgetting everything that was said is just too easy, especially when you're nervous. (When you find yourself getting nervous, take a few deep breaths to calm yourself down a bit.)

✔ **Insurance forms, cards, and other relevant data.** Many doctor's offices make copies of your insurance card and driver's license, and many billing departments won't file your claim unless you provide them with a form. Ask about what you need to bring before your appointment.

✔ **A list of any questions for your doc.**

Here are some questions you may want to ask your doctor:

- Why do you think I'm having these problems?

- If I don't have hypoglycemia, what do I have?

- When will you know what is causing the problem?

- What should I do now?

- What course of action do you plan on taking?

- What is the treatment plan?

- What diet plan do you recommend? (If your doctor says that nutrition has no bearing or that you simply need to eat a balanced meal, you're seeing the wrong professional. Find someone with more expertise in hypoglycemia.)

- Can you refer me to a nutritionist, dietician, or other alternative healthcare practitioner (someone other than a doctor who practices traditional Western medicine)?

In addition, coax a family member or friend into accompanying you on the visit. Bribe them if you have to; getting help is important. This extra person can prod your memory or provide more details about your illness, and he or she can give moral support to keep you on track if you get too nervous. (Or kick you in the shin if you're not making any sense.) Oh, one more thing: No visit to the doctor is complete without nutritional snacks and reading materials (or quiet hand-held computer games).

After the appointment, ask yourself these questions:

✔ Did I feel comfortable with the doctor?

✔ Did I feel comfortable asking questions?

✔ Do I have confidence in this doctor?

✔ Did the doctor spend enough time answering all my questions?

✔ Did I actually understand what the doctor was saying? Did he explain things in terms I understand?

If you weren't reasonably satisfied, visit another doctor. If you felt okay about everything, schedule a complete physical exam.

The complete exam will include tests for all your body's systems (cardiovascular, gastrointestinal, and more), as well as disease screenings. As you know, the doctor is going to take lots of things: a blood sample, urine and/or stool samples, and X-rays. Make sure to follow all instructions when preparing for the exam. If you're asked to refrain from eating or drinking anything other than water, do just as you're directed. If you don't follow your doctor's instructions, you can invalidate your test results.

Putting Some Ohhhhmm into It: Alternative Medicine

Two kinds of medicine can help relieve your hypoglycemia. We talk about one kind throughout this chapter: *allopathic medicine*. This conventional Western medicine targets specific illnesses with drugs and/or surgery. This type of medicine is actually ill-suited for addressing the chronic and numerous complaints of a typical low blood sugar sufferer.

However, you don't have to confine yourself to treatments by an MD. A health challenge is a health challenge. Today, patients can benefit from many acceptable alternatives. The American Board of Holistic Medicine (ABHM) defines *holistic medicine* as "the art and science that addresses the whole person, body, mind and spirit." The holistic approach to healthcare makes much more sense when treating hypoglycemia, because it focuses on the interconnectedness of body, mind, emotions, social factors, and the environment in determining the status of health. Only when these things are regarded as inseparable, with each affecting the others, is hypoglycemia effectively addressed.

 In addition to viewing the mind and body as inseparable, alternative medicines use *non-invasive* (not requiring surgery), *non-pharmaceutical* (herbal or homeopathic remedies instead of prescription drugs) techniques. Although these techniques aren't yet accepted by most conventional medical doctors, an increasing number of such doctors are beginning to offer both allopathic and holistic approaches.

More insurance plans are beginning to cover alternative treatment approaches, but even if your insurance doesn't cover the alternative therapy you choose, selecting an alternative medicine practitioner can be worth the cost.

Considering your alternatives

So what alternatives can you consider? The alternatives are too numerous to list them all here. Here are some that we believe may be especially helpful for hypoglycemia:

- **Nutritional counseling.** Because so much of the treatment for hypoglycemia revolves around food, we strongly recommend nutritional counselors who tend to concentrate on food's nutritional value and supplements that may be missing from your diet.

   Either a dietician or a nutritionist can do the job. It doesn't matter as long as the person is qualified and has a good track record of treating hypoglycemia. You can go to the American Dietetic Association's Web site (www.eatright.org) and find the names of registered dieticians.

- **Herbal medicine.** This alternative treatment involves using supplements, powders, and actual raw herbs. Basically, there are three major approaches to herbal medicine: Western, Indian (Ayurvedic), and Chinese. Just because something is natural, it doesn't mean that it can't also be dangerous. Remember, too, that certain herbs don't go well when taken with prescription medicine. Consult with your doctor before taking any herbal remedies.

- **Naturopathic medicine.** This type of medicine stresses health maintenance, disease prevention, and patient education and responsibility. It's not identified with any particular type of therapy; it's more a philosophy of life and health. You can find naturopathic doctors in your area by visiting The American Association of Naturopathic Physicians Web site (www.naturopathic.org).

- **Orthomolecular psychiatry.** This type of treatment is also called the *biochemical approach*. Orthomolecular psychiatry believes that when the brain is biochemically disorganized, so is the mind. It also believes that there are great individual differences in nutritional needs and metabolic processes. Doctors who practice this type of treatment use large, therapeutic doses of specific vitamins, nutrients, amino acids, trace elements, or fatty acids to achieve healing. They may also insist that you eliminate certain foods or food additives from your diet.

✔ **Acupuncture.** An acupuncturist inserts very thin, sterile, stainless steel needles into points along the body's meridians. (*Meridians* are invisible channels that form the body's energy network.) Many acupuncturists also use *moxibustion,* a procedure in which *moxa* (a dry, yellow, fluffy material made from the herb mugwort) is rolled into a cone or a tiny ball, placed on a meridian acupoint, and lit.

Acupuncture not only helps ease hypoglycemic symptoms but it may also address the underlying blood sugar problem. To contact a qualified acupuncturist, ask for recommendations from a trusted physician or friend. You can also visit the The American Academy of Medical Acupuncture Web site at `www.medical.org` for referrals.

Working in tandem

Combining the Western and Eastern methods of healing may create the best of all worlds. This combination of methods may sound like something that's not easy to accomplish, but it's actually quite possible. For instance, the clinics run by Dr. Chow (the co-author of this book) offer *integrated treatments* to patients. Patients get regular physical check-ups and conventional Western medical care, which includes prescription medication, but they can also receive chiropractic, acupuncture, and Chinese herb treatments. The doctor can recommend alternative therapies that are appropriate for the patient, or the patient may ask for integrated treatment. These one-stop clinics are becoming more common in larger cities. Ask your healthcare practitioner for a referral.

If you don't have the opportunity to go to a one-stop clinic, however, make sure that your alternative medicine practitioners work with your primary healthcare provider. This way, you can avoid getting conflicting advice or having an important aspect of your health overlooked.

Here's some additional advice to consider when you're being treated with alternative medicine:

✔ **Don't try too many different therapies.** It'll be confusing and very expensive for you.

✔ **Avoid doctor-hopping.** Make sure that you give one doctor and one approach sufficient time to work for you.

✔ **Create a file for yourself.** Keep an accurate record of all your office visits, meds, vitamins, supplements, and anything else that you've been given, and take notes at each session. Your healthcare providers should be aware of everything you're doing in terms of your health.

TIP

Releasing the qi with Chinese medicine

A growing body of research supports the benefits of traditional Chinese medicine (TCM). TCM particularly excels in conditions, such as chronic or nonspecific complaints, that Western medicine is weak at treating. All of TCM's practices are aimed at removing blockages to *qi* (or *chi,* which is loosely translated as "energy"), as well as at restoring, rebalancing, and increasing the qi of an affected organ or organs.

What can you expect from a visit to a practitioner of TCM? He will carefully examine your face and tongue, take your pulse, perhaps feel your abdomen, and ask you detailed questions about your health, diet, lifestyle, and so on before arriving at a diagnosis. The practitioner won't say that you're suffering from hypoglycemia. Instead, he may say, for instance, that there's too much dampness and cold in your body, and there's some stagnation in the kidney areas. In fact, two people with hypoglycemia can get different descriptions of what's ailing them, with the treatments varying accordingly. These differing diagnoses don't mean that the TCM doctors are wrong, or that what they're about to do doesn't have a prayer's chance of working. They simply mean that the causes of low blood sugar that are overlooked by Western doctors may be picked up by TCM practitioners, who view health through a different prism and attach different labels to dysfunctions of the body. Herbal formulas can be adjusted in infinitesimal ways to fit your body's constitution. Similarly, with acupuncture, needling techniques and points of insertion can be varied to suit your body's requirements.

With traditional Chinese medicine, some people see immediate improvement, while others do not. Realize that because TCM tries to get to the root of an illness, you may have to undergo many sessions before you see results. If you're interested in trying TCM, check your insurance plan to see whether it covers alternative healthcare. And make sure that the practitioner you visit is licensed and certified.

Part III

Getting Off Your Bleached-Flour Buns and Treating the Problem

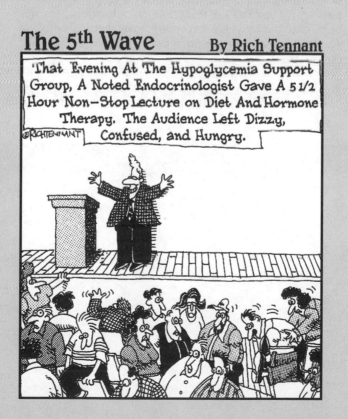

The 5th Wave   By Rich Tennant

That Evening At The Hypoglycemia Support Group, A Noted Endocrinologist Gave A 5 1/2 Hour Non-Stop Lecture on Diet And Hormone Therapy. The Audience Left Dizzy, Confused, and Hungry.

©RICHTENNANT

In this part . . .

*F*ood. It's everyone's favorite subject. In this part, we discuss the role of nutrition in health and, in particular, the great significance it has for the hypoglycemic person. We discuss the underlying biochemical disorder in chronic hypoglycemia. You discover that the only way you can recover from hypoglycemia is by changing your diet. Nothing else you do can have the same impact on your health. It doesn't matter how many flower essences you inhale, herbs or supplements you quaff, mantras you chant, or acupuncture treatments you receive: The bottom line is that you have to change your diet.

Chapter 6

Gorging on Good Health

● ●

● ●

*Y*ou may not know it yet, but the road to radiant health is paved with good foods. Granted, these foods may not be your number one preference right now, but as you make your way through this book, your palate and your taste buds will likely change.

Thankfully, treating hypoglycemia is directly linked to changing your diet. Vitamins and dietary supplements can help (see Chapter 7 for a complete list), but you don't need expensive medication to get results. Making changes to your diet does, however, take work and commitment. Only you can make the day-to-day changes required to turn your health around. But as you do so, you'll be heartened by the sense of vitality you experience as you recover from the lifestyle that made you ill. (For more on the concept of recovery, see Chapter 1.)

Creating a food plan that takes your biochemical individuality into account helps you achieve optimum health. Because each person has a unique *biochemistry* (no two bodies have exactly the same chemical characteristics and reactions), an optimal diet for one person may be inadequate for another person.

As you embark on your eating plan, try to think in terms of abundance rather than restriction and limitation. You'll undoubtedly have to give up some favorite foods, but you'll be replacing them with a wide variety of foods that you may not have tried before.

Depending on where you live, you may not find some of the foods mentioned in this chapter in regular grocery stores. They are, however, easily obtained in natural food stores or large, international grocery stores. If not, you can easily get them through suppliers over the Internet. See Chapter 17 for resources.

Of Food Pyramids and Healthy Eating

Do you often get strong cravings for something sweet or starchy: a candy bar, a bagel, mashed potatoes? (No, not broccoli. Who'd want that?) Your low blood sugar is driving you toward something that will give you a boost of energy. If you cave into your cravings, you can set off a chain of reactions that culminate in a *blood sugar crash* — when the blood sugar level falls below the optimum range in which the body functions.

The fact is that anything with white sugar and white flour is absolutely the worst food for blood sugar control. Here's what happens when you eat a carbohydrate-dense food (carbohydrate is starch, a class of food that includes bread, rice, and pasta): Your body releases more insulin. Insulin is like the messenger boy that goes from cell to cell delivering *glucose* (sugar) from the blood. But if you always have a lot of insulin hanging around, the insulin receptors on the cells become overwhelmed. Like surly teenagers, the cells soon stop responding. (For more on the role of carbs, see Chapters 1, 2, 3, and 4.)

Toppling the familiar pyramid

Many Americans try to eat healthy by eating a high-carb, low-fat, and low-protein diet. Part of the blame falls on the food pyramid recommended by the U.S. Department of Agriculture (USDA). You may have seen a picture of it.

At the base of the pyramid are grains such as rice, wheat, oats, and cereals. Six to eleven servings a day of this group are recommended. Moving upward, the next section features fruits (two to four servings) and vegetables (three to five servings). The third section has dairy products, meats, poultry, fish, eggs, dry beans, and nuts (two to three servings.). At the very top are the fats, oils, and sweets, which are to be consumed sparingly.

Over and low

For various reasons, low blood sugar can lead to weight gain.

✔ An increased desire for sweets, if indulged in, can lead to a weight problem.

✔ Overeating sweets and starches overstimulates insulin production. And too much insulin causes the excess storage of fat in the body.

✔ Hypoglycemics have a tendency to develop allergies. (See Chapter 6 for more on allergies.) These allergies can cause fluid retention, making it that much more difficult to lose weight.

Merely counting calories isn't enough if you want to lose weight. You need to ask yourself where the calories came from. From carbohydrates? Fats? Proteins? All of these sources are important considerations. The calories from a sliver of candy bar aren't the same as the same number of calories from a bushel of fresh vegetables. That's because vegetables are packed with fiber (candy bars have zilch in that area), which slows digestion and absorption, leading to better blood sugar control. (See Chapter 2 for more details.) As mentioned before, sugar creates an artificial appetite, which causes food cravings. Sugar can also cause mineral imbalances and digestive problems, resulting in an *allergy addiction* (an addiction to foods you're allergic to).

This diet is a no-no for the hypoglycemic person, because it can set off a yo-yo blood sugar syndrome. (You can partially offset this by eating enough fat and protein, but that may add up to way too many calories! Anyway, too many carbs aren't good for you.) Many people who go too low on fats and protein experience the following problems:

✔ Constant hunger

✔ Craving starch and sugar

✔ Deficiences in calcium and vitamins A, D, E, and K

✔ Liver's impaired ability to deal with toxins

To help stabilize your blood sugar, eat some protein with every meal or snack. (An exception to this rule is fruits. Some people experience digestive discomfort when they mix fruit with protein. Not everyone does, so experiment and see what works best for you.) Carbs affect your blood sugar the most, because they're easily digested and transformed into glucose. By contrast, protein is digested much slower. Eating some protein slows digestion and helps stabilize blood sugar. When it comes to your blood sugar, carbs really count. (A list of foods that contain protein is provided later in this chapter.)

Building a hypoglycemic pyramid

If you're hypoglycemic, and you want a healthy diet, just reshape the pyramid a bit as shown in Figure 6-1. Hypoglycemics have their very own food pyramid! At the base are fresh fruits and vegetables (more vegetables than fruits). The next section contains high-quality, low-fat protein (lean cuts of beef, skinless chicken). These two groups should fill up most of the pyramid. Dairy is there, just waiting for you to consume two to three servings. Near the top are the breads, grains, and pasta, which are to be seldom eaten. Fats and oils occupy the uppermost, narrow portion of the pyramid. The majority of your carbohydrate needs are met by fresh nutrient-dense fruits and leafy-green vegetables.

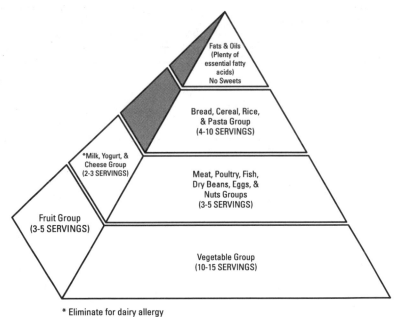

Fats & Oils
(Plenty of essential fatty acids)
No Sweets

Bread, Cereal, Rice, & Pasta Group
(4-10 SERVINGS)

*Milk, Yogurt, & Cheese Group
(2-3 SERVINGS)

Meat, Poultry, Fish, Dry Beans, Eggs, & Nuts Groups
(3-5 SERVINGS)

Fruit Group
(3-5 SERVINGS)

Vegetable Group
(10-15 SERVINGS)

* Eliminate for dairy allergy

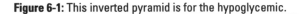

Figure 6-1: This inverted pyramid is for the hypoglycemic.

If you use this hypoglycemic food pyramid as your guide, keep the following things in mind:

- ✔ Carbohydrates should comprise 40 to 60 percent of your total calories. Nutritionally speaking, it's much better to eat complex carbs (whole wheat bread) than simple carbs (white bread). But before you go on an eating spree of all-organic, all-natural, whole-wheat cakes and breads, consider this: Even complex carbs have the tendency to raise your blood sugar and trigger excess insulin production. Restrict your total carbohydrate intake.

- ✔ Protein should comprise 15 to 30 percent of your total calories. Remember, though, that while protein occupies a significant portion of your diet, it should by no means outstrip your carbohydrate intake. Aim for regular and consistent protein intake, not a high protein intake.

- ✔ Unless your doctor has put you on a special diet, you should strive to get about 15 to 20 percent of your calories from fats.

Keeping your diet in balance

The key to using the modified food pyramid is keeping things balanced. Here are some clues that you may be getting too much or too little of the different food groups and what you can do to fix the situation.

Too much protein, too few carbs

Depending on body size, the maximum amount of protein a person can tolerate is about 200 to 300 grams a day. If you experience the following symptoms, you're most likely eating too much protein and not enough carbs:

- ✔ Nervousness
- ✔ Irritability
- ✔ Jitters
- ✔ Overall feeling of weakness
- ✔ Compulsion to overeat

If you do experience these symptoms, they'll most likely clear up a few days (several weeks at most) after you add carbs to your diet.

Too much protein can pose these health problems:

An ongoing debate

Whether the traditional pyramid truly reflects a foundation for a sound diet remains a matter of debate. The plan has drawn fire from circles that base their criticism on recent studies of human nutrition. For instance, one such study indicates that our daily requirement for whole grains may not be as vital as our need for fresh fruits and vegetables. Experts remain divided on what constitutes a healthful diet. So what are you, the consumer (and you truly are consuming!), supposed to do? You can't stop eating until a firm conclusion is drawn!

Fortunately, you don't have to wait for a final verdict before picking up your fork. Almost everyone agrees on certain points, such as avoiding junk food. (Sorry to say, but everyone agrees that the human organism doesn't require chips and fries to function properly.) Data drawn from experiments suggests that hypoglycemics do better when they avoid a heavy concentration of starches and sugars.

- ✔ Damage to the liver, kidneys, and brain
- ✔ Calcium deficiency
- ✔ Gouty arthritis (a painful condition of the joints caused by excess uric acid in certain tissues)

Too little fat (believe it or not)

Americans and people in many other Western countries may be paying lip service to the much-publicized low-fat diet, but if industry sales of high-fat ice cream are any indication, people are still letting quite a bit of fat slip through their lips. Although too much fat is unhealthy, in general, fats

- ✔ Help your body function properly
- ✔ Slow down the rate at which carbs enter your bloodstream
- ✔ Give you the satisfying sensation of being satiated
- ✔ Release a hormone that signals your brain to stop eating

If you're hypoglycemic and you don't consume enough fat (about 15 to 20 percent of your diet), you may start craving starches and run the risk of eating too much.

Shunning problematic foods

Food not only has the ability to make you sick but it can also heal. In the case of hypoglycemia, the key to successful treatment is

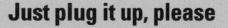

Just plug it up, please

Did you know that in the 1800s white bread was used to treat diarrhea? Refined carbohydrates such as white bread are devoid of fiber. Lack of fiber causes constipation. Without fiber, foods pass through the digestive tract slowly, festering in the colon and serving as food for harmful bacteria that produce gas and toxins. White bread was used as a kind of plug for the colon. You may want to remember this the next time you're tempted to reach for that white dinner roll your waiter serves you!

Besides, eating the bread rolls that restaurants often serve before meals is especially hazardous. Eating pure carbs on an empty stomach virtually guarantees that your blood sugar will drop too low. In response, you'll be tempted to eat more bread — with the same unfortunate result. Besides, bread is very light but high in calories. When you're feeling hungry, bread doesn't fill up your stomach quite as quickly as other foods that have more fiber and nutrients. So you have to eat a lot of bread to feel satisfied.

through the elimination — not the addition — of certain foods. Avoiding foods that wreak havoc on your system has the greatest impact on your health — as much (or more) impact than what you eat or what supplements you take.

This section includes a list of foods and beverages that you should avoid. After you've followed this outline for a while and your body becomes stronger, you can expand your diet and even "cheat" occasionally. When you're transitioning to a healthier diet, be as careful as possible. If you usually inhale the typical Western diet, many familiar foods (perhaps your all-time favorites) may be included in the huh-uh list. Don't despair, though. You don't have to follow the recovery program perfectly for it to work.

These are the foods that you should shun:

- ✔ Sugar (includes white, brown, raw, and turbinado).

- ✔ Refined flour (white, bleached, unbleached, and enriched flour) and everything made from it. Generally speaking, if it looks white, it's white flour! Read labels, avoiding anything not made from whole grains.

- ✔ Polished rice (white rice).

- ✔ Processed proteins (lunchmeats, sausages, bacon, hot dogs — anything with additivites or preservatives).

> ✔ Processed cheese (cheese made by combining one or more natural cheeses with an emulsifying agent, and then heating and mixing it; American cheese is processed).
>
> ✔ Coffee, black tea, and anything else with caffeine (includes chocolate).
>
> ✔ Soft drinks (carbonated drinks, including all colas).
>
> ✔ Alcohol.

The World's Your Oyster and Your Mango — Foods to Eat

After checking out the list of foods to avoid, you may be feeling that you're forced to make the grim choice of either never enjoying eating again, or living out the rest of your life in compromised health. In fact, you don't have to do either.

Eating a wide variety of foods — within the constraints of your hypoglycemic diet — ensures that you're getting the proper balance of vitamins and minerals (which are discussed in depth in Chapter 7).

Most people today are so chock full of artificial foods and flavors, that they forget that healthy food is also truly good-tasting food. You can eat lots of delicious foods; moreover, when you embark on your recovery program, unhealthy foods start losing their appeal. Although you may always hear the siren call of your favorite forbidden foods, it will become more muted over time; besides, you'll have so much more zest for life, that you'll want to get right back on course.

Life's a bowl of cherries: Fruits

Fruits are yummy, not to mention rich in nutrients and all kinds of beneficial compounds. And they're just the thing to eat if you want something sweet.

The sugar in fruit is called *fructose,* and it appears that fructose doesn't cause as rapid a rise in blood sugar as simple sugars. Fructose has to be changed to glucose in the liver before it can be used by the body, so the rise in your blood sugar is more moderate when you eat fruits. Besides, fruits can help control sugar cravings (instead of triggering them, as processed snacks do.) But don't consume fructose alone, without the fruit, because then it's almost as bad as table sugar.

The preferred fruits for hypoglycemics are of the not-too-sweet variety:

- Apples
- Cherries
- Pears
- Strawberries
- Kiwi
- Mango
- Papaya
- Guava
- Grapes

Fruits to avoid, especially while you're in the initial stages of recovery, include the following:

- Bananas
- Figs
- Dates
- Raisins and other dried fruits (unless eaten in small amounts after soaking in water or cooking with cereal)

Ideally, all the fruits and vegetables you eat should be organically grown, as conventional fruits have been sprayed with pesticides that some people are sensitive to; hypoglycemics tend to be more susceptible to toxic overload. If you can't get organic produce, or you find that it's too costly, use fruit and vegetable washes to rinse out most of the chemicals. You can get these washes at health food stores. Or, alternatively, add a teaspoon of bleach to 3 quarts of water, and soak the produce in it for 15 minutes.

Vegging out isn't a bad thing

Your mother was right: You need to eat your veggies. Do you want to be free of distressing hypoglycemic symptoms? Eat your vegetables. Do you want to combat aging and look and feel young for as long as possible? Eat your vegetables. Do you want your brain to remain sharp, clear, and focused? Eat your vegetables. Vegetables carry a greater nutritional wallop than most man-made vitamins or supplements. They're chock full of vitamins, minerals, protein, high-quality carbs, essential fatty acids, antioxidants, fiber, and a host of other health-promoting substances that scientists are only beginning to unravel. (The green parts of plants are rich in essential fatty acids, especially the they're-so-darn-good-for-you Omega-3 oils.) If we were fully appreciative of the power-pack vegetables have to offer, describing someone as "a real vegetable" would be considered a compliment.

The USDA recommends three to five servings of veggies daily, but most people eating the typical Western diet fail to meet this all-too modest quota. The minimum should actually be 8 servings, but, ideally, you should eat anywhere from 10 to 15 servings. If your diet consists mainly of wilted lettuce, mashed potatoes, and overcooked or canned vegetables, or if you think ketchup is a vegetable, you're in for a culinary surprise. Try opening your taste buds to a cornucopia of delights with the dark and leafy greens, and the vivid reds, oranges, yellows, and purples. (The brightly colored ones contain more *antioxidants,* substances that protect you from the free radicals that damage cells.)

Always try to eat fresh vegetables in their raw state, because cooking destroys some of the nutrients. On the other hand, some vegetables, such as asparagus, cauliflower, and cabbage, may promote better digestion when lightly cooked. Raw spinach can interfere with calcium absorption, so if you do eat it raw, make sure that you don't consume it with calcium-rich foods. For variety, you can

Darned if you do, darned if you donut

Donuts and danishes spell disaster when it comes to your blood sugar. Muffins (even if they're low fat) and bagels, which seem to be healthy alternatives, will spike your blood sugar just as high and just as rapidly. This is also true for breakfast cereals (if you're going to eat sugar-coated cereal, you may as well have a candy bar) and *muesli,* a Swiss breakfast cereal consisting of rolled oats, nuts, and fruits.

Health food stores carry all sorts of cereals that actually contain some good vitamins, but these, too, are best avoided, especially in the early days of your recovery. If you do eat these types of cereal, make sure that you choose the ones that have no added sugar of any sort, no additives, and lots of fiber. Slow-cooked oatmeal is a healthy choice, particularly if you throw in some crunchy protein-rich nuts or seeds. (Steer clear of instant oats and other instant foods, which convert almost instantly into blood glucose.) *Steel cut oats* — the inner portion of the oat kernel — are best. They contain more nutrients, because they're less processed than quick, instant, or rolled oats. Steel cut oats, which are also called Scotch oats or Irish oatmeal, are chewier, have more texture, and are slower to cook. They're available at health food stores.

steam, sauté, stir fry, bake, boil, or grill your veggies. Just be careful not to cook the life out of them. (See recipes and serving tips in Chapter 15.)

You can eat the following veggies in their raw form as often as you like:

- Celery
- Cucumbers
- Iceberg lettuce
- Romaine lettuce
- Parsley
- Watercress
- Bell peppers
- Radishes
- Turnips

Other veggies vying for your attention include

- **Garlic and onions.** These veggies are of special interest to hypoglycemics and diabetics because they contain special sugar-regulating factors. They also reduce LDL cholesterol ("bad" cholesterol) and lower blood pressure. See *Controlling Cholesterol For Dummies,* by Carol Ann Rinzler (Wiley Publishing), for more information on managing your cholesterol.

- **Avocados.** This vegetable helps lower your cholesterol levels. People who are watching their weight tend to stay away from avocados, but the fats are good for you, and the sugars do not stimulate insulin production. It seems, in fact, that they suppress insulin production — a boon for hypoglycemics. Diabetics, on the other hand, should exercise some caution.

- **Artichokes and string beans.** These vegetables are excellent for both the hypoglycemic and the diabetic. Artichokes improve blood circulation and mobilize energy reserves. However, they contain 10 to 14 percent carbs, so eat about a quarter of a whole one, and never more than one a day. String beans contain an insulin-like hormone and work as a sugar balancer.

- **Sprouts and sea vegetables.** Sprouts make good convenience foods, as they're easy to grow, they're inexpensive, and you can throw them in many dishes, such as soups and salads, to suit your taste. If you want to grow sprouts, you can buy the seeds at health food stores. Kelp can be used in soups or for making stock, and sheets of seaweeds (like the sheets of nori that sushi rolls are wrapped in) are both handy, versatile, and rich in trace minerals. Make sure that you buy unsweetened seaweeds. They're available in most health food stores and Asian markets.

The squeaky hypoglycemic gets the grease: Fats

Fats have gotten an undeservedly bad rap in recent years. Too much of the wrong kind of fats (saturated) is bad, but we do need fats (unsaturated is best). Without them, we'd suffer from nerve damage and other afflictions.

- ✔ Saturated fats: These "bad" fats are found in red meat and high-fat dairy products.

- ✔ Unsaturated fats: These "good" fats are found in things like nuts.

 The best way to get good fats is to drizzle flax oil on your salads, eat fatty, cold-water fish like salmon, and eat avocados. You needn't worry about getting too much fat if you're eating lean meats. The excess fat in most people's diets comes from junk food.

Fats you need

In order to function properly, the body needs *essential fatty acids* (EFAs). They're *essential* because they have to come from outside sources — the body can't manufacture them. The long-chain Omega-3 fats from fish and fish oil are particularly beneficial, but they're woefully deficient in the modern diet. Cold-water fish, such as salmon, trout, tuna, and sardines, provide abundant sources of Omega-3 fats. You can also get them from flaxseed oil, chopped walnuts, or eggs that have been enriched with Omega-3.

 Olive oil is one of the healthiest mass-produced oils. It appears to aid proper sugar metabolism, making it good for hypoglycemics. Make sure that you use the real thing — extra virgin olive oil, not light virgin. Similarly, if you use sesame seed oil, get it unrefined and untoasted.

Fats you don't

 While too much saturated fat may be bad, trans fatty acids and altered vegetable fats are extremely destructive and should be totally avoided. Transfatty acids are artificial fatty acids that block the natural fatty acids. Margarine and many processed snack foods contain these trans fats. (Read the labels and stay away from them.)

Fats such as margarine and shortening are created through a process called *hydrogenation,* which hardens the oils and gives them a longer shelf life but destroys their essential nutrients. Some fats are partially hydrogenated, which also produces trans fatty acids. The irony is that many people switched from butter to margarine in an erroneous effort to protect their hearts. So butter up with the real thing — or better yet, eat as the Italians do and dip your bread in olive oil.

Powering up with proteins

Eat some protein at every meal. It ensures slow sugar absorption and helps prevent hypoglycemic symptoms. We're not talking about a huge amount of protein, however, just a regular, consistent intake to help balance your blood sugar.

The preferred protein sources for hypoglycemics are

- Nuts (macadamia, hazelnut, walnut)
- Seeds (flax, sesame, pumpkin)
- Nut butter (also Tahini and sesame butter)
- Eggs (from free-range chickens)
- Fish and seafood
- Chicken (with the skin removed)
- Turkey (with the skin removed)
- Game meats (rabbit, venison, buffalo, game birds)
- Organ meats (chicken and beef liver)
- Lean meats (organic meats; occasionally pork, if at all)

Meat in the middle (of your whole-wheat bread)

Organic meat comes from livestock raised without hormones and antibiotics. As mentioned, antibiotics can precipitate hypoglycemia, and hormones may have adverse effects on your health and are better avoided. You can find organic meat at health food stores. If you can't find any health food stores near your home, check out the Web sites in Chapter 17. (Of course, if you buy organic meat, you can't just cook it any way you want. Deep frying it or coating it with white flour won't do your hypoglycemia much good.)

Whaddaya, nuts?

Nuts and seeds provide high quality protein in addition to EFAs, minerals, fiber, and vitamins E and B-complex, which protect against stress and are involved in mechanisms for blood sugar control. (Chapter 7 has more on minerals and vitamins.)

Perhaps you're afraid to eat nuts because you're concerned about weight. If so, the results of a study of a large group of Americans should put your mind at rest. The study showed that the people who ate the most nuts tended to be less obese (probably because the high amounts of fat and protein in nuts produce a feeling of fullness). Of course, no one is suggesting that eating as many nuts as you want all day long is going to lead to weight reduction!

You can eat two to three servings of nuts per day. One serving is roughly ten whole almonds or peanuts, six walnuts, or two pecans. One serving of seeds is about one tablespoon.

Make sure that the nuts or seeds are not rancid. Choose ones without cracks, stains, or splits. And never, under any circumstances, eat nuts or seeds that are moldy. Try to purchase them unshelled, raw, and unsalted. If you have to get them shelled, buy whole nuts (not crushed or slivered). Keep them in the fridge and eat them fresh.

Doing dairy

Don't consume more than 2 to 3 servings of dairy per day. Eliminate it completely if your hypoglycemic symptoms are severe. Livestock are given antibiotics, which get into the dairy products and encourage the growth of yeasts and fungi that can precipitate allergies, sugar cravings, and hypoglycemia. You can resume eating modest amounts of dairy products after your condition has stabilized.

Breaking the proverbial camel's back: Breads and grains

Carbohydrates are of great interest to hypoglycemics — and diabetics — as they bear the greatest impact on blood sugar level. Eating the right kinds of carbs in the right amounts is critical in blood sugar management.

Carbohydrates can be either simple or complex.

✔ **Simple carbs** — such as sugar, refined flour, and white rice — are essentially sugars, and they spike your blood sugar rapidly. Simply put, simple carbs are the worst foods for blood sugar control. That's why we have to say that sugars fall into the ugly category of foods that do more harm than good.

✔ **Complex carbs** take longer for the body to break down into glucose, and therefore they deliver sugar steadily, making it more likley that blood sugar will be stabilized. For the hypoglycemic, this point can't be overemphasized. Whole grains and legumes are complex carbs.

Whole grains and legumes are complex carbohydrates. Refined grains have their germ and bran removed, which partially or totally eliminates at least 36 nutrients. Whole grains, by contrast, retain these nutrients.

Whole grains include the following:

✔ Brown rice

✔ Whole wheat

✔ Buckwheat

✔ Unpearled barley

✔ Whole oats

✔ Unhulled millet

✔ Quinoa

✔ Amaranth

Legumes provide two to four times as much protein as grains. They also help improve liver function and blood sugar control. They include

✔ Black eyed peas

✔ Chickpeas

✔ Garbanzo beans

✔ Kidney beans

✔ Lentils

✔ Lima beans

✔ Pinto beans

Aye, aye, GI

The *glycemic index* (GI) ranks carbohydrates by the effect they have on blood sugar levels. To get a fair idea of whether a particular food has a high, low, or intermediate GI ranking, remember that

✔ The longer you cook a food, the higher its GI

✔ The more processed a food is, the higher its GI

✔ The less fiber a food has, the higher its GI

Scientists developed the GI to help diabetics choose the best carbohydrates and better manage their blood sugar. Before developing the GI, doctors and nutritionists treated most starches as interchangeable. But to everyone's surprise, fruits such as grapes, which are considered rather sweet, were found to cause less of a blood sugar rise than plain white bread.

Today, many books and Web sites offer a fairly comprehensive listing of the glycemic index of foods. With a mixed meal (foods with different GIs), calculate the average of the indexes of all the carbs you're going to eat. If you choose individual items that are lower in GI, the overall index for your meal will be lower. (This is one way you can ease yourself into eating a low-carbohydrate diet.)

To give you some idea of the speed at which sugars from different types of foods enter the bloodstream, a list of a few common foods is provided in the following table. Bear in mind that, for any given food, different sources will give a slightly different GI. Foods with an index of 70 or more are considered to have a high GI, foods with an index from 50 to 69 have an intermediate GI, and foods with an index below 50 have a low GI.

One more factor to consider is the *carbohydrate density (CD)* of a food. Calculate it with the following formula:

total carbohydrate – fiber content = the amount of digestible carbs (CD)

A high level of CD can stimulate too much insulin production, with a consequent drop in blood sugar. So although complex carbs such as whole grains are good, you should limit yourself to about two servings per day. Your body will function best if most of your carbs come from non-starchy vegetables.

Glycemic Index (GI) of Some Common Foods

Breads	GI score	Breads	GI score
pita	57	whole wheat	72
rye	60	bagel	72
white	72	melba toast	100

Cereals	GI score	Cereals	GI score
oatmeal, slow cooked	46	cream of wheat	66
muesli	58	corn flakes	83
oatmeal, instant	66		

Fruit	GI score	Fruit	GI score
cherry	22	kiwi	52
plum	24	mango	55
grapefruit	25	papaya	58
strawberry	32	banana	62
pear	36	raisin	64
apple	38	cantaloupe	65
peach	42	pineapple	66
grape	43	watermelon	72
orange	43	dates, dried	103

Grains	GI score	Grains	GI score
barley	24	couscous	65
whole wheat	43	millet	74
buckwheat	54	white rice	86
brown rice	59	instant rice	120

Legumes	GI score	Legumes	GI score
soybeans	18	chickpeas	36
kidney beans	27	navy beans	38
lentils	30	pinto beans	42
butter beans	31	baked beans	43
split peas	32		

Snacks	GI score	Snacks	GI score
sponge cake	46	blueberry muffin	59
fruit bread	48	bran muffin	60
ice cream, regular fat	50	soda crackers	106
pound cake	54	jelly beans	114
Danish	59		

You can find grains and legumes in natural food stores. They're often sold in bulk, so you can easily find the right ones by just looking at the labels — or by asking a store clerk. (If you can't find them in bulk, look for them in packages or cartons with labels.)

Because carbs have a profound effect on your blood sugar level, you need to choose your carbs as wisely as you choose your friends. Whenever possible, choose complex carbs over simple carbs. If you're ever in a situation where you have no choice, or if you have an irresistible urge to eat sugary food, see the Cheat Sheet at the front of this book before making any other moves.

Eating Patterns, Serving Sizes, and Other Healthy Stuff

You're ahead of the game if you're familiar with serving sizes. Fear not if you haven't a clue what a serving platter is (much less a serving size). We lay out the game plan for you in this section, helping you figure out serving sizes and when to eat.

Eating six squares a day

The good news is, being hypoglycemic means never having to say you're hungry. That's because you get to eat three small meals and three snacks (or six small meals if you prefer) at two to three hour intervals. The object is to ensure that your blood sugar never drops too low. Even if you don't have much of an appetite, you shouldn't let too many hours go without eating — except when you're sleeping.

The most important meal

A blood-sugar balanced day begins with a good breakfast. You want to eat shortly after you wake up, preferably within an hour, and definitely not longer than two hours.

If you're in the habit of exercising and/or meditating for more than an hour before breakfast, take some protein powder before your workout to prevent a blood sugar drop. If you don't, you may be tempted to gobble down anything that gives you instant energy. (*Protein powder* is a concentrated form of protein that you can drink like a shake. Read labels to make sure that the protein powder you choose doesn't have any added sugars. You can get powdered whey protein or soy protein at health food stores or on the Internet. See Chapter 17 for resources.)

Don't feel like having breakfast? In that case, incorporating exercise into your morning routine will virtually guarantee that you'll be ready — even ravenous — for food. Even if you can't exercise in the morning, following a regular hypoglycemia eating plan gets your body accustomed to eating shortly after waking up.

Sizing up your servings

When you're sticking to a healthy diet, you need to watch your serving sizes (for information on how much of what you should get at a meal, see "Of Food Pyramids and Healthy Eating," earlier in this chapter). You don't have to measure your foods precisely: You're not conducting a chemical experiment! You probably won't be able to stick with a diet that requires you to accurately weigh or measure everything you eat. Besides, you'd look pretty silly if you pulled out a scale or a calorie counter when eating out.

Think of 1 serving as roughly

- 1 slice whole grain bread
- ½ cup oatmeal or other cooked whole grains
- 1 cup carrots
- ½ cup beans, peas, or lentils
- ½ cup corn
- 1 small apple, orange, or pear
- 1 medium peach or nectarine
- ½ banana
- ½ cup pineapple
- ¼ melon

To familiarize yourself with what a serving size is, measure some foods you eat. That way, you'll have a visual estimate of how much you're eating. According to the American Dietetic Association (ADA), most people overestimate serving sizes. (Just some wishful thinking here!) Table 6-1 offers the ADA's helpful visual comparisons for estimating one serving size.

Table 6-1	Estimating a serving size
Food	*What a serving size looks like*
Cooked lean meat, poultry, or fish (2–3 ounces)	An audiocassette or personal digital assistant
Cheese (1.5 ounces)	Four stacked dice
Fruit, cooked vegetables, cooked rice or pasta	Tennis ball cut in half
Raw leafy vegetables	Tennis ball

Here's an easy way to figure out how much protein to get: Make a fist with either hand. Take a good look at it. The size of your fist is the amount of protein you should get at each meal. In other words, the meat on your plate should be no larger than your fist. Don't worry about the serving sizes of your non-starchy veggies: You can eat as much of those as you like. You'll never get a carbo overload from leafy green vegetables. You can eat up to 5 servings a day of starchy vegetables (such as carrots).

A few other notes for beginners

When you begin your hypoglycemia eating program, you're better off limiting fruits to two servings a day. As your condition improves, you can eat four to five servings a day. A serving is one small orange or apple. However, if you have a strong craving for sweets, and you feel like you're going to break down and gorge on forbidden pastries (like a double fudge chocolate cake), grab a fruit — even if it means exceeding your daily quota.

Exercise caution with the carbs from bread, cereal, rice, and pasta. When you begin your dietary program, you can get faster results by completely eliminating this group. After a month or two, you can reintroduce them into your diet. Even then, limit this food group to no more than four servings per day — two servings a day, ideally. If you start experiencing hypoglycemic symptoms, cut back immediately.

The following list provides a guide to the food categories and proper ratios of consumption that will best serve your hypoglycemic diet. As a general rule, your meals should include the following:

- Protein should comprise 15 to 30 percent of your total calories.

- Carbohydrates should comprise 40 to 60 percent of your total calories.

- Fats should comprise 15 to 30 percent of your total calories.

As a general rule, aim for 30 percent protein, 40 percent carbs, and 30 percent fats early in your program. As you progress in your recovery, cut back on protein and increase your consumption of carbs. Do so gradually, noting any reappearance of symptoms.

If you stick to your food plan, by the end of the third or fourth month you should be generally clear of all hypoglycemic symptoms. (Again, bear in mind the individual differences between people.) At this time, you should be eating 15 percent protein, 60 percent carbs, and 25 percent good fats.

One-third to one-half of the fats in each meal should be in the form of essential fatty acids, and you should have at least 50 grams of dietary fiber a day. (For more about fats, see "The squeaky hypoglycemic gets the grease: Fats," earlier in this chapter.) You may start out on the higher end of the fat and protein consumption guidelines when you embark on the program for recovery and then gradually begin cutting back.

This dietary plan is for hypoglycemics. If you're diabetic, be vigilant about serving sizes and food exchanges. For more information, see *Diabetes Cookbook For Dummies,* by Alan L. Rubin, MD (Wiley Publishing).

Soybean Burgers Are Your Bag, Baby: Vegetarians

So you skip the animal flesh. No eggs or dairy, either? You have to make sure that you get enough protein and avoid eating too many grains and carbohydrates. A traditional source of protein is legumes (such as beans and lentils), which were known as "the poor man's meat" in the early part of last century. You should be aware, however, that they are much higher in carbohydrates than protein, so they should be supplemented with other protein sources; at the same time, you need to go easy on eating other forms of carbs so that you don't get a carbo-overload.

If you're not a strict vegetarian, fish can be an excellent way to complement your diet. If you don't eat fish, make sure that you get enough essential fatty acids by taking fish oil capsules or flaxseed oil. Walnuts are also good sources of EFAs. You may also add an occasional egg or natural cheese. If you're concerned about cruelty to animals, look for eggs from *free-range chickens* (ones that aren't cooped up).

Foods such as tofu (bean curd) and tempeh (cheeselike cooked beans) are extremely versatile, and you can make literally hundreds of dishes with various forms of soy. Be sure to check the labels when buying imitation meat products such as soy hamburgers, because some brands contain more carbs than protein. Remember, even too much of a good thing can compromise your health, so try not to lean too heavily on soy. Be sure to eat a wide variety of foods.

Chewing on the Idea of a Food Journal

No two people have exactly the same biochemistry. Research on biochemical individuality has shown that requirements for each essential nutrient can vary tenfold or more. With that in mind, you can see how a diet that may work for someone else may not work as well for you. Therefore, for best results, you need to customize your dietary plan.

We detail the most crucial dietary customization steps earlier in this chapter; you should follow those steps before molding the plan to your own body.

Keeping a daily food journal is the backbone of your recovery process and of personalizing the general plan. The object of the food journal is to help you see exactly what you're doing. It helps you become aware of the foods and beverages you're consuming. With a journal, you can start to see the connection between what goes into your mouth and your moods, feelings, and bodily sensations.

Find a notebook that you like and feel comfortable using. You can get a regular notebook, or you can purchase something that is constructed of handmade paper or bound in leather. If you prefer, carry around large index cards or loose paper and then staple them together at the end of the week. Make sure that you write the date clearly on each card. You can also use a micro cassette

recorder; if you do, we still recommend that you transcribe everything down onto paper at the end of the day (or several days).

When you keep your daily food journal, make sure that you write
down the following things:

- ✔ Exactly what you eat and drink
- ✔ What exercises you engage in
- ✔ Your feelings, both physical and emotional
- ✔ Anything else that seems relevant (you may also want to add
  comments)

The journal will

- ✔ Keep you focused and aware of what you're eating and drinking and how you're feeling. It will help keep you on track.

- ✔ Prevent you from engaging your mental auto-pilot and consuming foods unconsciously. If you park yourself in front of
  the TV, it's very easy to eat a bag of chips or guzzle down an
  entire six-pack without really being aware of what you're
  doing.

- ✔ Help you pay attention to yourself. It may even be the first
  time in your adult life that you've taken the time to do so. As
  you continue to write in your journal, you'll begin to discover
  your own needs and rhythms. You may be so accustomed to
  taking your cues from others outside of yourself — your parents, your peers, television commericals — that perhaps
  you've forgotten how to listen to your own body.

Don't worry if you forget to write things down, or if you don't know
how to explain your feelings. Gradually, you'll become adept at recognizing your feelings. It's important to accept whatever you're
feeling without blaming or criticizing yourself.

Writing down any physical or emotional changes you may be experiencing is especially important. For instance, if you have more
energy or you're unusually irritable, be sure to note it. Instead of
jotting down your feelings only after you eat, make a point of writing them down every hour or two. Recording your feelings can
make it easier to see how certain foods (or combinations of foods)
affect your mood or physical symptoms. You don't have to write
lengthy essays, just a word or two will suffice.

When you write what you are feeling on a regular basis, you may
begin to uncover

✔ Connections between foods that you never suspected before

✔ Whether a recurrent feeling is triggered by something you eat or by the stresses in your life

✔ What's working or not working in terms of your diet

✔ Where and how you drifted from your eating program (if you did drift; what are you, superhuman?)

The more you know about what's going on with yourself, the easier it is to make any necessary adjustments in your life. Highlight your journal, and circle any links you see. Have fun while becoming your own private investigator.

Look over your journal every week. If you can, look it over on the same day of the week (Sunday, for example) so that you don't forget. After you start identifying the patterns and feeling more confident about your food choices (perhaps in a month or two), you can review every two weeks. But if you notice anything unusual (like the appearance of certain symptoms), don't wait to refer to your journal.

Keeping a daily food journal helps you make refinements and get better results. On the other hand, avoid straying too far from the basic recommendations. You'll know when you aren't following your diet correctly, because your hypoglycemic symptoms (see Chapter 3 if you need a refresher on symptoms) will reappear. Don't sweat it if they do; just get right back to following your healthy eating plan.

Chapter 7

Hanging with Herb and His Buddies Vitamin and Supplement

Should you or shouldn't you take vitamin and mineral supplements? The next time you're bored in a meeting or at a social gathering, bring up this question. Add to the discussion a disorder that some people argue doesn't even exist, and there you have a fine debate.

Although dietary therapy is the cornerstone of hypoglycemia treatment, anyone suffering from blood sugar imbalance has an increased need for many nutrients that aren't easy to obtain only from food. Nutritional supplements handle many symptoms as well as help improve blood sugar control.

This chapter shows you how to use herbs, vitamins, and minerals to address specific hypoglycemic symptoms and discomforts. Chapters 8, 9, and 10 show you additional ways you can cope and survive — even thrive — with this metabolic disorder.

Getting Acquainted with Herb

When you get to know "Herb," you find that he's a pretty interesting fellow. He's been around for a very long time, and he's been all over the world. Yes, herbs have probably been used since the dawn of humankind, and herbal medicine is no passing fad.

Traditionally, people in Europe, India, and China have relied on herbal medicine to prevent and heal illnesses. Some evidence shows that even nonhuman primates have used herbs for healing.

Humans have learned to treat a variety of complaints — from insomnia to allergies — through herbal remedies. In some cases, *herbs* (roots, flowers, and other parts of plants with medicinal properties) can be just as effective in treating some common ailments, if not more so, than prescription and over-the-counter medications; they're generally safer, too.

This effectiveness in treating ailments does not mean, however, that herbs are completely safe. Just because something is natural, it doesn't mean that it's completely without side effects — some substances can be "naturally poisonous," after all. Also, before combining herbal treatments with prescription medications, check with your physician and an experienced herbal practitioner.

As long as you use herbs as instructed and take them in the right doses, they have a good safety record. Some herbalists warn that certain herbs or formulas taken for a long time can lead to toxicity. So don't continue to take something for longer than you need, and take breaks from the products. Keep in mind that these are just general guidelines; everyone reacts to herbs differently. What works for your Aunt Ninny may not work for you.

Saying Hello to Supplements and Vitamins

Not only did Mom tell you to eat your veggies but she also made you down those big, nasty-tasting vitamins. Who knew she was right about that, too?

Most everyone knows the word supplement, but do you know what a *supplement* is? They're nutrients, such as vitamins and minerals, that you add to your regular diet in the form of pills, powders, or liquid.

It's a good practice to sometimes give your body a break from the vitamin pill, because your body can become habituated to them, decreasing their effectiveness. By stopping from time to time, you'll still enjoy the benefits of supplementation while reducing the costs. One way to do it is to take vitamins for one month straight and then go off them for a week. Or you can take them for six days and break for one day.

Vitamins and minerals

Vitamins, which are vital to the regulation of *metabolic processes* (chemical changes in living cells by which energy is provided) are generally classified as being

- ✓ **Water soluble.** If they're water soluble, they're not stored in the body. Any excess gets flushed into the urine — this is why some doctors insist that all you get from taking vitamins is expensive urine.

- ✓ **Fat soluble.** This type of vitamin is stored in the body, so be careful not to take too much. They can build up to a toxic level. The fat soluble vitamins are A, D, E, and K. Some doctors discourage supplementation, because they're afraid that people will be careless and take too much. This isn't usually a problem, unless you're taking megadoses for an extended period of time.

The American Medical Association and the National Academy of Sciences continue to maintain their official stance by saying that there are no benefits to supplementation as long as you are eating a proper, well-balanced diet. Yet there's a large and growing body of evidence that suggests that significant health benefits can be gained from taking vitamins. Many medical doctors are beginning to recognize that vitamins and minerals, often in amounts that would be difficult to get through food alone, can alleviate certain conditions.

For more information on vitamins, see *Vitamins For Dummies,* by Christopher Hobbs, LAc, and Elson Haas, MD (Wiley).

Supplements

Nutritional *supplements* are vitamins in the form of tablets, capsules, powders, or liquids, and they can be natural or synthetic. *Natural vitamins* are derived from natural sources — from plant or animal tissues — while *synthetic vitamins* are created artificially to assume the same chemical structure as the natural vitamin.

Choose natural vitamins whenever you can, because they may contain substances, that scientists are not necessarily aware of, that may provide extra benefits. Besides, the substances found in natural vitamins remain in their natural ratio, which works better. Synthetic vitamins may also have added artificial colorings and flavorings that you're better off without. Always read the labels to make sure that they contain no added sugar, yeast, or preservatives. The label tells you if the vitamin is natural or synthetic.

You should never let taking supplements be an excuse for eating poorly. Aim to get as many nutrients as possible from actual foods.

Taking the Hypoglycemia Mix

Table 7-1 lists the daily vitamins that nutritionists and practitioners have found to be beneficial to the health of people suffering from hypoglycemia.

Please note that the dosages listed in the table are guidelines. The recommended dosage levels may vary with one's age, activity level, and current nutritional status. You can easily get the recommended levels by taking a multiple vitamin and mineral formula (for resources on where to buy them, see Chapter 17) and then adding specific nutrients that may be missing or that aren't provided in high enough amounts.

Although they're higher than the RDA (Recommended Daily Allowance), the following dosages are not considered megadoses, and taking them should not result in any unwanted side effects. However, it's always best to consult your primary care physician or healthcare practitioner before you begin any regimen of supplements.

All the ingredients in supplements should appear on the label. The amounts in Table 7-1 are given in milligrams (mg), micrograms (mcg), and international units (IU).

Table 7-1	Vitamins and Minerals That Can Benefit Hypoglycemics If Taken Daily	
Vitamin	*Amount Per Day*	*Benefit*
Vitamin A (acetate)	5,000 IU	Maintains healthy skin and good eyesight; treats acute infections.
Vitamin A (beta carotene)	10,000 IU	A double-vitamin A molecule that the body can eliminate.
Vitamin C	2,000 mg	Supports the adrenal glands.
Vitamin D	200 IU	Helps body absorb and use calcium.
Vitamin E (d-alpha tocopheryl acetate)	400 IU	Prevents degenerative diseases of the cardiovascular, neurological, and respiratory systems.

Vitamin	Amount Per Day	Benefit
Thiamine (Vitamin B1)	100 mg	Crucial for a healthy nervous system Important for adrenal glands and converting glucose to energy.
Riboflavin (Vitamin B2)	50–100 mg	Crucial for a healthy nervous system. Helps regulate mood.
Niacin (Vitamin B3)	100 mg	Crucial for a healthy nervous system. Important for adrenal glands and converting glucose to energy.
Niacinamide (Vitamin B3)	50–75 mg	Crucial for a healthy nervous system.
Pantothenic acid (Vitamin B5)	1,000 mg	Crucial for a healthy nervous system.
Pyridoxine (Vitamin B6)	50 mg	Crucial for a healthy nervous system. Deficiencies in Vitamin B6 are sometimes linked to hypoglycemia.
Vitamin B12	400–1,000 mcg	Crucial for a healthy nervous system. Important for adrenal glands and converting glucose to energy.
Biotin	300 mcg	Important in food metabolism. Plays essential role in production of fatty and amino acids.
Folic acid	400–1,000 mcg	Important in the metabolism and use of protein and amino acids.
Mineral	**Amount Per Day**	**Benefit**
Boron	1–2 mg	Helps the bones use calcium. May also help regulate calcium, magnesium, and phosphorous balance.
Calcium	1,500 mg	Metabolizes sugar.
Chromium	400 mcg	Essential for insulin function and metabolizing carbohydrate.
Copper	1 mg	Helps in the healthy functioning of nerves and joints.
Iodine	75 mcg	Helps the thyroid control metabolic rate and body temperature.

(continued)

Table 7-1 *(continued)*

Mineral	Amount Per Day	Benefit
Magnesium	750 mg	Important for metabolizing sugar.
Manganese	10 mg	Helps utilize vitamin C and some B vitamins; facilitates glucose metabolism.
Molybdenum	50 mcg	Helps metabolize carbohydrates.
Potassium	200 mg	Supports electrical impulses across cell membranes. Assists in body's energy use.
Selenium	200 mcg	Functions as part of the body's detoxifying systems. Important in cancer prevention.
Zinc	50 mg	Plays crucial role in glucose and insulin regulation.

The following vitamins and minerals should be taken in *divided doses,* so you don't take the entire dose at once. In other words, if you're taking 1,500 mg of calcium a day, you can take 500 mg in the morning, 500 at noon, and 500 in the evening. For some people, taking too high a dosage of pantothenic acid can cause diarrhea; taking a smaller dosage several times a day prevents this problem.

- ✔ Calcium
- ✔ Magnesium
- ✔ Vitamin C
- ✔ Thiamin
- ✔ Niacin
- ✔ Vitamin B12
- ✔ Pantothenic acid

In addition to taking the previously mentioned vitamins and minerals daily, you may want to include the supplements described in Table 7-2. They're particularly helpful because they support glucose and insulin metabolism, facilitate glands involved in blood-sugar regulation, raise blood sugar levels, and/or enhance mood. Who doesn't love an enhanced mood?

Table 7-2	Supplements That Can Benefit Hypoglycemics If Taken Daily	
Supplement	*Amount Per Day*	*Benefit*
L-glutamine. Do *not* take if you have Reye's syndrome, cirrhosis of the liver, or kidney problems.	1 gram on an empty stomach.	This amino acid (which is most abundant in the body) raises blood sugar levels and reduces fatigue. Also energizes the brain and maintains a healthy digestive system.
L-tyrosine. Consult your doctor before taking if you have lupus. Do *not* use if you're taking MAO inhibitors.	1 to 2 grams.	This amino acid enhances mood and facilitates adrenal, thyroid, and pituitary functioning.
CLA (Conjugated linolenic acid)	3,000 to 4,000 mg	This natural fatty acid supports the healthy metabolism of glucose and insulin.

Symptoms and Their Salient Supporters

Now we get to the fun part: symptoms! Fortunately, you can summon stalwart supporters to your aid. We list some of the most common symptoms of hypoglycemia and things you can take to alleviate them.

You're not going to have all of the symptoms listed in the following sections, and even though the symptoms are associated with hypoglycemia, it's possible to have one or more of them despite not having the disorder. If you want to know more about the symptoms of hypoglycemia, flip to Chapter 3.

See your primary care physician before starting a supplemental program. In addition, when you consult with any healthcare practitioner, always let him know exactly what supplements you're taking.

Anxiety

Are you anxious about everything? Are you just plain anxious about nothing in particular? Have a kava kava. This herb will help you relax but remain alert. (People are more prone to feeling aches and pains when they're suffering from anxiety.) Kava kava contains active ingredients that are thought to work like aspirin. Look for it in *tinctures* (highly concentrated liquid herbal extracts) and capsules at herbal shops.

You should not take kava kava if you're pregnant or nursing, and you should never take more than the recommended dosage listed on the product labels, unless directed to do so by a healthcare practitioner. Also, be aware that if you take alcohol or barbiturates, kava kava will have a stronger effect on you.

Some other supplements are good for helping control anxiety. Be careful not to take the following supplements at night: They can be too stimulating, making it hard for you to sleep.

✔ **Skullcap.** This herb, which contains minerals such as calcium, iron, potassium, and magnesium, revitalizes the nervous system. It's good for easing stress, anxiety, and depression, as well as alleviating premenstrual syndrome. Use as an extract.

✔ **Passionflower.** This herb is especially effective if you have anxiety attacks in the middle of the night. You can brew passionflower into a tea (steep two teaspoons of the dried herb for 30 minutes in a cup of freshly boiled water), or you can consume it in a tincture. Don't use passionflower for more than two weeks.

✔ **GABA (gamma-amino butyric acid).** This amino acid and neurotransmitter can be found in capsule form. Take the recommended dosage described on the product.

✔ **Vitamin B.** You should make sure that you're getting enough vitamin B. Studies on both humans and animals suggest an association between anxiety and deficiencies of vitamin B complex. Take 25 to 100 mg of vitamin B complex a day, as a single dose or in *divided doses* (the required dose split into 2 or 3 doses).

✔ **Inositol.** This vitamin-like substance is often grouped with the B vitamins. A study showed that its effects are similar to those of mild tranquilizers. *Therapeutic doses* (amounts high enough to have a medicinal effect on the person taking it) of inositol range from 500 to 1,000 mg per day. In some sensitive individuals, too high a dose can cause diarrhea.

If you have recurrent, long-standing anxiety problems that aren't caused by medical conditions, you should definitely make meditation, deep breathing, and relaxation exercises a part of your daily life. (Chapter 10 helps you do that.) Because anxiety and depression often go hand in hand, you may want to refer to the sections "Depression/mood swings" and "Stress," later in this chapter.

Asthma

People who suffer from asthma have labored breathing that is often accompanied by wheezing, coughing, or gasping. They may experience a sense of constriction in the chest.

The following supplements can help reduce the severity of asthma attacks, however, you should not, under any circumstances, substitute these remedies for what your doctor prescribes you. In case of a serious attack, call your doctor or go to the emergency room.

- ✔ Garlic works as a mucus regulator for chronic bronchitis. Garlic cooked with chicken soup is especially nourishing. Inhaling the fumes while the soup is cooking can help alleviate asthma symptoms. Sip the soup throughout the day.

- ✔ Fish oil capsules are beneficial. The oil should be from fish high in anti-inflammatory omega-3 fatty acids (salmon, mackerel, sardines, and tuna). You'll have to take these capsules for 10 weeks or so before you'll start noticing benefits. Avoid fish oils if you're allergic to fish.

- ✔ The Indian spice turmeric is also a good anti-inflammatory agent. The whole spice itself, however, isn't potent enough to do the job. Instead, get capsules that contain curcumin, and take at least 400 mg a day.

- ✔ Nettle (the root juice or leaves) can help relieve asthma symptoms and allergies. Some very potent ginger extracts naturally reduce inflammation throughout the body.

Chronic fatigue syndrome

If you have hypoglycemia associated with chronic fatigue syndrome, the following supplements may provide some relief:

- ✔ **Echinacea.** Good for fighting colds, flu, and infections; boosts the immune system in general.

- ✔ **Siberian ginseng.** Useful in fighting stress and fatigue. Protects the liver and helps prevent memory loss. Boosts energy.

- **Ashwaganda root.** Energizes by nourishing the kidneys.

- **Ginkgo biloba.** Improves circulation, sharpens memory, reduces anxiety, and boosts concentration.

- **DHEA (dehydroepiandrosterone).** Improves neurological function, immune function, and stress disorders.

- **Hydrocortisone.** Used in the treatment of chronically stressed and weakened adrenals.

- **NADH (nicotinamide adenine dinucleotide).** It's found in all living cells, and it's essential for their development and energy production. Helps fight fatigue.

- **SAM-e (S-adenosyl-methionine).** It's an amino acid derivative that's normally synthesized in the body. Some evidence suggests that it may be a fast-acting, safe, and effective antidepressant.

- **Licorice.** No, not the candy! Don't take this supplement if you have high blood pressure. Licorice has anti-inflammatory, anti-allergic, and anti-arthritic properties.

- **Astragalus.** Strengthens the immune system by helping the body produce antibodies and working in the bone marrow to produce white blood cells.

Constipation

Who hasn't suffered from constipation at one time or another? Thanks to the modern diet, it's become a common problem in the so-called civilized world. Just staying away from sugar and refined flour should soon relieve (indeed!) your problem. The following remedies may help relieve constipation:

- Allicin, a substance found in garlic, stimulates the contractions of the intestinal walls. Eating garlic by itself can upset your stomach, so you may want to stir fry it with onions or mix it with yogurt to help buffer it. You never know, this new flavor of yogurt — vanilla with crushed garlic cloves at the bottom — may just become the next big rage at your local supermarket.

- Eating radishes can help alleviate constipation, too. Radishes in yogurt may be interesting, but they'll probably taste better in a salad.

- Try eating whole grain barley products (the less processed, the better).

If you've had chronic problems with constipation, or if you haven't produced a bowel movement for a week or longer, you should go see your doctor.

Depression/mood swings

After you stabilize your blood sugar, your depression should begin to ease (unless underlying problems exist). If you're hypoglycemic, make sure that you follow the recommended dietary changes in this book or the changes outlined by your healthcare practitioner. That alone should make a significant difference. At any rate, with all the pharmaceutical, vitamin, and herbal aids out there, not to mention psychotherapy and counseling, no one should continue to suffer the debilitating effects of depression.

People with clinical depression should seek professional help immediately. If you've been feeling blue for more than a couple weeks, get help. (See Chapter 10 for a more complete treatment for depression.)

Here are some supplements that can help elevate your mood and even out your highs and lows:

- ✔ **Vitamin E.** This supplement can reduce mood swings. Make sure that you take the natural form, d-alpha (d'l-alpha is the synthetic form). The recommended dosage ranges from 400 to 1,600 IU (international units) daily. If you're diabetic or you have bleeding problems, you should talk to your physician before taking vitamin E in dosages over 100 IU.

- ✔ **Selenium.** This supplement is an essential mineral that should be taken with vitamin E. Selenium makes vitamin E work better, and medical trials have shown that it improves mood.

- ✔ **Folic acid.** People with a dietary deficiency of folic acid, part of the B vitamin complex, exhibit depressed mood, lethargy, poor concentration, and irritability. But studies suggest that taking folic acid supplements can help even if people aren't deficient. It seems to aid the response to antidepressant drugs, even in people who were previously unresponsive to medication. For some people, folic acid by itself may be enough to relieve depression. Take 500 mcg daily.

- ✔ **Acetyl L-tyrosine.** Positive effects have been noted with acetyl L-tyrosine. Take 1,000 to 2,000 mg daily on an empty stomach. Higher doses should only be taken under doctor supervision, because they can raise your blood pressure or lead to rapid pulse. Do *not* take acetyl L-tyrosine with MAO inhibitor drugs, or if you tend to suffer from migraines.

✔ **L-tryptophan.** This amino acid is highly recommended by leading health experts. It helps the body increase its production of *serotonin,* the feel-good neurotransmitter that's often low in depressed people. Blood levels of tryptophan are also usually low in depressed people.

Take 2 to 4 grams of L-tryptophan daily. Take it before bedtime on an empty stomach. It works best if you also take niacinamide. Do *not* take tryptophan if you have asthma, because it can make your breathing problems worse.

✔ **SAM-e (S-adenosyl-methionine).** Some evidence suggests that SAM-e (pronounced "Sammy") may be a fast-acting, safe, and effective antidepressant. It's an amino acid derivative that's normally synthesized in the body. It starts working in a week or two (sometimes in just a few days), compared to 2 to 6 weeks for prescription medication. People in Europe have been taking it for depression for years. Unlike medication, SAM-e doesn't come with a laundry list of side effects.

Start by taking one 200 mg tablet in the morning on an empty stomach. (Take it with food if it upsets your stomach; it won't work quite as effectively with food, so you may need to take a larger dose.) You can gradually increase the dosage up to 1,600 mg, depending on your needs. Generally, 400 mg seems to work. Be sure that the tablets are *enteric-coated,* otherwise your body won't absorb them properly. (Because the special coating can withstand stomach acid, enteric-coated tablets dissolve in the small intestine for maximum absorption.) Studies have shown that taking folic acid, B12, and B6 will give you even better protection against depression. Do not take SAM-e too late in the day, as it may interfere with your sleep.

✔ **NADH (nicotinamide adenine dinucleotide).** This *coenzyme* (active form of an enzyme system) plays a pivotal role in our body's energy production and can be safely combined with SAM-e. Start with 2.5 mg daily and increase your dosage by 2.5 mg each week until you find the right dose for you.

You should not take NADH too late in the day, as it can overstimulate you and prevent you from sleeping. Take it first thing in the morning on an empty stomach.

✔ **St. John's Wort.** This supplement, which was widely used in Europe before gaining popularity in the United States, has received a lot of media play for its antidepressant effects. It's good for mild to moderate depression. You need to take it for four to six weeks or longer before starting to see any beneficial results. Make sure that you take capsules standardized to 0.3 percent hyperium. St. John's Wort may cause sensitivity to the sun.

Some other random helpers: Black cohosh reduces mood swings, anxiety, and depression, and hot flashes in postmeno-pausal women. Damiana is supposed to be good for depression and anxiety, also. Take it three times a day as an *infusion* (herbal tea) or tincture. Sip dandelion tea if you think suppressed anger is causing your depression.

Digestive problems

You started eating the right foods, but your GI tract is throwing fits anyway. What can you do?

Stomach

Many digestive problems are caused by eating the wrong foods, as well as by eating them in far too large a quantity. As you eat less of the foods that made you sick in the first place and turn to the rec-ommended hypoglycemic diet (see Chapter 7), your digestive system will stop getting so overburdened.

Until this change in diet helps your condition improve, you can take licorice capsules before meals. (Please do not confuse this supplement with licorice candy, which will do you no good!) Taking two or three capsules about a half an hour before meals can pre-vent heartburn.

Digestive enzyme supplements can also help improve digestive problems. Choose those that can facilitate the digestion of protein, fat, carbohydrates, fiber, and milk lactose. The enzyme capsules should include pancreatin, amylase, protease, lipase, and amylase.

Liver

When it comes to digestion, there's one organ that you probably haven't considered: the liver. It's an underappreciated organ that slaves away each day, detoxifying your blood and ridding your body of poisonous substances. It's responsible for more than 500 functions. Secreting bile to aid in fat digestion is just one of these many functions.

When you have indigestion, it's not necessarily your stomach that's upset: It's often your liver. Well, you'd be upset, too, if no one ever thanked you for the all the work you do!

The least you can do is to give your liver some assistance. Here are some supplements to help you out:

- ✔ **Barberry.** Bitter compounds in barberry stimulate digestive function. Barberry can also help fight infections and stomach problems.

- ✔ **Elderflower.** This herb assists with digestion. It's also good for coughs, sore throats, fever, and hay fever.

- ✔ **Peppermint.** Herbs in the mint family are excellent for digestion. Peppermint stimulates bile flow and the secretion of digestive juices.

- ✔ **Gentian.** This bitter herb increases the numerous secretions along the entire digestive tract and helps get digestion back on track.

- ✔ **Milk thistle.** This herb has an active ingredient that's one of the strongest known liver protectors. It prevents toxins from damanging liver cells and speeds the healing of any damage to the liver.

- ✔ **Dandelion.** This herb aids digestion.

- ✔ **Turmeric.** This bitter herb forms the base of most Indian curries. It's good for digestion, it helps build the blood, and it eases menstruation. It contains ingredients that are anti-inflammatory, antioxidant, and liver-protective.

Now it's not exactly an herb, but the artichoke plant is also good for improving digestion and liver function. The part that's beneficial is the large basal leaf (everything but the heart). Clinical studies show that the basal leaves are good for digestion and liver function — what the studies neglect to mention is that they're also really delicious! Of course, it may be hard to eat an artichoke every day, even if you like them.

A convenient way to enjoy the benefits of artichokes is to take an artichoke extract. (Black radish juice extract also encourages the liver to produce bile.) You can take 300 to 600 mg of standardized artichoke extract before, during, or after a meal. If you eat six small meals a day, though, you don't need to take the extract at each meal. Just take the extract whenever you need to, such as when you end up eating more than you want to. You should refrain from taking artichoke extract if you have gall stones or an obstruction of the bile duct.

Fatigue and energy drain

Fatigue is something everyone experiences, especially if they have low blood sugar. A general feeling of fatigue is not the same thing as Chronic Fatigue Syndrome (CFS). A diagnosis is critical but, generally speaking, you may have CFS if you have severe, unexplained fatigue that's not relieved by rest and that lasts for at least six or more consecutive months. (For more on CFS, see Chapter 3. For supplements that can help relieve the symptoms of CFS, see "Chronic fatigue syndrome," earlier in this chapter.)

For run-of-the-mill tiredness, you can try the following supplements.

- ✔ **Mint.** Herbs in the mint family can help revive energy.
- ✔ **Lemon balm.** This herb calms, soothes, and revives energy.
- ✔ **Stinging nettle.** This herb is good for anemia, as it contains iron. It can also help with midafternoon slumps.
- ✔ **Oatstraw.** This herb is a tonic that can relieve both physical and emotional fatigue. It's a good supplement to take when you're feeling frazzled and exhausted.
- ✔ **Potassium.** This supplement is known to enhance energy and vitality. Take potassium aspartate with magnesium asparate.

- ✔ **Acetyl L-tyrosine.** This supplement is an amino acid. Take 1,000 to 2,000 mg daily. Do *not* take acetyl L-tyrosine if you're taking MAO inhibitor drugs or if you tend to suffer from migraines.
- ✔ **NADH (nicotinamide adenine dinucleotide).** This supplement is known as the "energizing coenzyme." It plays a crucial role in producing energy. With regular supplementation, you can expect to enjoy more energy and improved athletic performance. For instructions on dosage, see "Depression/mood swings," earlier in this chapter.

If you suffer from fatigue, be sure to rule out any possible medical causes. People with hypoglycemia sometimes have thyroid problems, so get your thyroid checked before trying the more potent herbs, such as Siberian ginseng, which can boost your energy but may be too strong if you have a weak constitution. Get a *standardized extract,* which ensures that you're getting the standard potency and tells you the exact amount of the ingredient. The dosage level depends very much on your condition. You may have to take the Siberian ginseng for several weeks before you feel an appreciable difference. When you take ginseng, avoid caffeine and other stimulants.

Fibromyalgia

Fibromyalgia is estimated to afflict between 6 and 12 million people in the United States alone. It's a painful, debilitating syndrome that affects mostly women and bears a striking resemblance to chronic fatigue syndrome. Some people with hypoglycemia may also suffer from fibromyalgia. For more on fibromyalgia, see *Fibromyalgia For Dummies,* by Roland Staud, MD, and Christine Adamec (Wiley).

Intravenous vitamin and mineral injections may produce a significant improvement in the symptoms of fibromyalgia. For this type of treatment, you need to consult a knowledgeable physician. The periodic use of UltraClear or UltraInflam detox programs, which are available through physicians, have also been known to help relieve the symptoms of fibromyalgia.

SAM-e, which is an anti-inflammatory that helps relieve muscular pain, and NADH (see "Depression/mood swings," earlier in this chapter) are also beneficial for treating the symptoms of fibromyalgia. If your condition is severe, you may want to try a 1 gram dosage of SAM-e daily.

Headaches

Headaches are yet another common symptom that hypoglycemics often experience. Migraines can sometimes be triggered by a bout of low blood sugar. If you get headaches halfway between meals, it may be the result of having too much insulin in your bloodstream — which then leads to hypoglycemia.

You may be able to alleviate your headaches with the following remedies:

- Fish oil capsules are beneficial for the prevention of headaches. Unless you're allergic to fish, you should eat more cold-water fish, such as salmon, mackerel, and trout. If you're pregnant, avoid fish unless otherwise instructed by your doctor.

- Ginger prevents the release of substances that make blood vessels dilate. Keeping blood flow even can help prevent and relieve migraines. Use fresh or powdered ginger when you cook. You can also grate fresh ginger into juice.

- Feverfew is a popular garden herb with anti-inflamatory properties that are beneficial for both arthritis and migraine headaches. Feverfew may help keep blood vessels from constricting, which can stop a throbbing headache. It stimulates the uterus, so don't use it during pregnancy.

- Mullein eases many kinds of lung ailments and strengthens the respiratory tract.

You should see a doctor if correcting your blood sugar imbalance does not help relieve your headaches, or if you have recurrent and/or severe headaches.

Insomnia

Everyone needs some good, restful Z's. If you don't get them, you're bound to be listless, unfocused, and crabby. Inadequate or poor-quality sleep counts as *insomnia,* an underdiagnosed and undertreated sleep ailment. Insomnia can be a short term (a single night to a few weeks), intermittent (episodes occur from time to time), or chronic (occurs most nights and lasts months or more) condition. If you suffer from insomnia, it may be caused by a serious illness, so don't wait to go to your friendly doctor.

If your insomnia is not caused by an underlying illness, or it's one of the symptoms of your hypoglycemia (and you should get a proper diagnosis for that, too), here are some things that can help:

- ✔ Try taking calcium along with magnesium at nighttime (in a ratio of 2 to 1). Take anywhere from 150 to 800 mg per day. Don't rely on milk alone, because it won't provide you with the correct amount of calcium.

- ✔ Inositol, a relative of the B-complex family, has a calming effect and encourages sound sleep. For temporary insomnia, take 500 to 1,500 mg at bedtime. (Don't take any other B-complex vitamins at bedtime, because they may keep you awake.)

- ✔ Tryptophan, taken before bed, has a calming effect. Don't take tryptophan if you have asthma.

- ✔ Kava kava and valerian are helpful for preventing insomnia. One study suggests that valerian root improved sleep for 80 percent of people with sleep problems.

- ✔ Some people find that drinking lettuce juice helps them sleep better.

Niacin (B3) may be helpful if you fall asleep easily but can't go back to sleep after waking up in the middle of the night. Take 25 to 100 mg a day. You may experience a *niacin flush* (where you feel overheated and your face begins to redden) in the first few minutes after taking it. If you notice these flush symptoms, decrease your dosage or take *no-flush niacin,* which doesn't cause flushing.

Low sex drive

Garlic breath may not exactly be an aphrodisiac, but eating garlic will stimulate the hormone glands, which, in turn, will rev up your sexual powers. Are you interested in finding out more? Men will be eager to hear that garlic stimulates the central nerve of the penis and helps cause an erection. Garlic will also nourish and strengthen your entire body, giving you the stamina to romp a little longer in the hay.

The health-conscious Chinese use a lot of garlic in their cooking. (Come to think of it, maybe that's why they have a problem with overpopulation!) The Koreans eat a lot of garlic, too, and a low birth rate isn't one of their problems. Anyway, try garlic in your cooking and take garlic capsules so that you can maintain a consistent intake.

Nettle and red clover are also said to be good for the libido. And for women, damiana is reputed to amp up sexual interest when sipped before bed. (But why restrict it to bedtime?) It's also supposed to alleviate depression and anxiety, two conditions that can dampen one's sexual appetite. Take damiana three times a day as an infusion or a tincture.

The Chinese regard the kidneys as the fountain of energy, and the kidneys and adrenal glands as the seat of sexuality. Take daily doses of angelica, dang gui, ginseng, chasteberry, and saw palmetto as tinctures to help your kidneys and adrenal glands function smoothly. Saw palmetto has been shown to be as effective in reducing the size of a man's prostate gland as the prescription medication Proscar. Anything that will *tonify* — balance and strengthen — the kidneys is good.

Memory problems/poor concentration

The following supplements can help improve your memory and concentration:

- ✔ **Choline.** The brain needs this substance to produce a major neurotransmitter.

- ✔ **Pantothenic acid.** Like choline, it's needed by the brain to facilitate the transmission of impulses between neurons.

- ✔ **Gingko tablets.** Gingko leaf extracts contain antioxidant properties. They also improve memory and alertness, and show promise in treating Alzhemier's disease.

- ✔ **Gotu kola.** Evidence indicates that gotu kola energizes the brain and improves concentration. Herbalists sometimes call this plant a vitamin for the brain.

- ✔ **Rosemary tea.** It's a handy-dandy way to perk you up anytime you're feeling dragged out. Drinking this tea is also a good way to start out the morning. Come to think of it, it's a good way to end the day, too.

Nausea

Ginger works well for nausea, motion sickness, morning sickness, and dizziness. It quells an upset stomach, reduces cholesterol, and strengthens the heart's overall functioning. For related conditions, see "Digestive problems," earlier in this chapter.

Mid-afternoon slump

It's all too easy to grab some coffee and a sweet roll to help you get out of the afternoon doldrums. The caffeine and sugar duo — a double whammy — may perk you up, and you may even think that you're more productive; but don't kid yourself, you're only setting yourself up for a blood sugar crash to rival Black Monday's stock market crash. You'll be blue, and you'll be sorry, as you pay dearly for the teensy bit of indulgence. It's not worth it, especially when there are so many healthy alternatives.

For instance, you may want to try

- **Dandelion root tea.** This herb balances blood sugar and helps support liver function.

- **Yerba mate.** This South American herb is a great antioxidant that elevates mood and alertness without giving you the jitters.

- **Stinging nettle.** This popular mineral tonic is rich in vitamins and minerals. It can help heal inflamed mucous membranes caused by colds and coughs.

- **Ginseng.** This revered root is a good adrenal tonic that boosts energy. It's especially popular for increasing vitality and sexual energy. It also improves functioning of the lungs and stomach and of digestion.

- **Gotu kola.** This herb accelerates the healing process, boosts memory, eases anxiety, increases energy, and protects against stress.

- **Reishi.** This red mushroom strengthens the immne system and calms the nervous system. It can also help regulate blood sugar. It's often prescribed for general weakness and fatigue.

- **Grapefruit oil.** This supplement acts as a brisk refresher. It boosts memory and increases energy and mental ability. You can get it in teas, tinctures, and capsules.

Poor circulation

Are you an ice princess or prince because of poor circulation? Remember to exercise regularly, as exercise (more than anything else) helps improve your circulation. Chapter 8 can get you moving in the right direction. In addition, you may also want to try the following:

- ✔ Eat more garlic. (So what doesn't garlic do?)

- ✔ Add ginger to your cooking, or grind it up and steep it as tea. Ground ginger in bottles is okay for cooking and flavoring, but it's generally not potent enough for healing purposes.

- ✔ Eat warming foods, such as healthy soups. Drink your beverages at room temperature or warmer. (Try to avoid iced beverages.) Refrain from eating raw vegetables until your body becomes *hotter* — when it's stronger and circulation has improved. In traditional Chinese medicine, people with a weak constitution who tend to suffer from cold hands and feet are told to avoid eating raw vegetables because they have a cooling effect on the body. Instead of eating cold salads, try quickly steaming your salads — for only a minute or two, so as not to destroy the nutrients. Rather than eat fruits or yogurts straight from the fridge, leave them out for a while so they're not ice cold to the touch. (But don't leave them out so long that they become spoiled.) Making sure that food doesn't spoil is especially important in the summer.

- ✔ Sprinkle ground cinnamon and cayenne pepper into your socks and gloves (they should preferably be made of cotton) to increase circulation and help warm cold hands and feet.

Be careful not to get cayenne in your eyes! Wash your hands thoroughly before touching yourself — or anyone else. If your skin is sensitive, don't touch the pepper with bare hands.

Stress

When it comes to vitamins, supplements, and herbs, just about anything that improves your overall health or strengthens the functioning of any organ will help combat stress.

An anti-stress vitamin regimen should include the B-complex vitamins, vitamin C, vitamin E, magnesium, calcium, potassium, chromium, manganese, selenium, and iron. Specifically, keep the following supplements in mind (and mouth):

- ✔ **Pantothenic acid.** This vitamin is required for the adrenal glands to work properly. If you're very stressed, take more than 700 mg daily in single or divided doses.

- ✔ **Pyridoxine (vitamin B6).** This vitamin helps with the synthesis of the neurochemicals important for counteracting stress. Don't take more than 100 mg, however, because excessive doses can cause nerve damage. It's also best if you take it with the same dosage of other B-complex vitamins.

- ✔ **Mugwort.** This herb, available in liquid or tea form, is often prescribed for stress. You can take it as a tincture or place a half ounce of dried herb in half a cup of water. Use caution if you have hay fever or are allergic to hazelnuts. Stay away from this herb if you're pregnant or on blood thinners.

- ✔ **Ginseng.** This famous herb will help you adapt to just about any physiological stress. It helps restore equilibrum when your body has been thrown out of whack by stressors. Siberian ginseng provides an enhanced overall physical endurance. Korean ginseng is good, too, but its effects may be a little too potent.

- ✔ **Reishi mushrooms.** These mushrooms are an excellent tonic. They give you a sense of overall well-being. You should refrain from taking too many of these mushrooms, especially if you are still young, as their effect is very strong. As with anything, you need to find a good balance.

- ✔ **Astral.** This herb is also a good tonic. It supports the immune system and helps the adrenal glands deal with stress.

You may also want to consider the relaxing herbs, such as the popular chamomile, lavender, valerian, lemon balm, passionflower, hops, and California poppy.

Water retention

You may experience water retention as a result of your hypoglycemia (or for a variety of other reasons).

If water retention is so severe that pressing on a swollen spot leaves indentations on your skin, go see your doctor immediately. Otherwise, you may want to try one of the following remedies to help relieve your discomfort:

✔ **Try some diuretic herbs.**

  • Corn silk tea is a safe and effective diuretic. But don't sip it at night, because it'll make you go to the bathroom.

  • Nettle and dandelion also have diuretic properties.

✔ **Drink more water.** Water can help relieve water retention, especially if you also cut back on sodium.

Taking a Whiff: Aromatherapy

Because the *limbic system* (which includes the brain's hypothalamus, hippocampus, and amygdala; the limbic system is especially concerned with emotion and motivation) processes both odor and emotions, smells evoke powerful and immediate reactions in us. *Aromatherapy,* using essential oils for therapeutic purposes, can be a good addition in soothing hypoglycemia's laundry list of physical and emotional effects, and smoothing your transition to a healthier lifestyle.

Essential oils are the aromatic and volatile liquids derived from herbs or plants. Because essential oils are highly aromatic, you can get many of their benefits by simply by inhaling or diffusing them into the room. Buy only pure, natural essential oils if you want the full range of physical and psychological benefits of aromatherapy.

After you get used to handling the oils, they're quite safe. But as with anything, including prescription medicine, they need to be treated with precaution. When it comes to essential oils, be aware of the following don'ts:

✔ Do *not* take essential oils by mouth, as they can be quite toxic. If you accidentally swallow an essential oil, call your local poison control center (it's good practice to keep the number in a handy place) or 911 immediately.

✔ Don't get the oil in your eyes or on other sensitive parts of your body.

✔ Don't let children or pets near essential oils. Keep the oils out of their reach.

✔ Don't ever apply any of the essential oils directly to your skin without first diluting them. The oils are very concentrated, and they will irritate your skin.

✔ Don't forget to consult a knowledgeable healthcare practitioner before using any essential oils. If you suffer from serious or chronic illnesses, such as cancer, epilepsy, heart disease, or asthma, be very careful about using essential oils; their potency is nothing to sniff at.

If you have very sensitive skin or a lot of allergies, do a patch test before using an essential oil. Dab a two-percent solution of the essential oil and water on a small patch of skin, such as the under-side of your arm. Over the next 12 hours, check to see if there's any redness or itching. If there is, do not use the oil on your skin. Even if you can't apply the diluted oil to your skin, you can still dab it on a tissue, hankie, or cotton ball and inhale it as needed. You can also put a few drops in your bath.

If you really want to get into aromatherapy heavy duty, several books on the subject are available, including *Aromatherapy For Dummies,* by Kathi Keville (Wiley Publishing). You can also find out more from a reputable aromatherapist. Ask for referrals for trained, certified aromatherapists from people you trust.

Rocking Bach's Flower Remedies

This is true flower power! The theory behind flower remedies is that the energy of flowers contained in *flower essences* (the extract from flowers) treat emotional patterns that result in the manifestation of physical symptoms. One of the most popular formulas, Bach's Rescue Remedy, is reputed to be quite effective for stress. Some people even use them for their pets. For Web sites, see Chapter 17.

Right now, virtually no scientific studies back up the claims of flower-essence healing, mostly because the essences don't lend themselves readily to scientific research. So, although they're fun to try, be careful and controlled in your experiments, and know that essential oils and flower essences cannot replace advice from a doctor. When in doubt, always consult a healthcare practitioner.

Chapter 8

Easing Symptoms and Energizing with Exercise

· ·

· ·

*P*ower. That's the last thing you feel when your body and brain cells aren't properly fueled. What's more, as a hypoglycemic you've probably been chronically undernourished, so the weakness lingers. You must balance your blood sugar to properly fuel your body.

Unfortunately, you can't balance your blood sugar and properly fuel your body by using a quick fix; permanent lifestyle changes are the only way to go. Changing your diet is the first step. Chapter 6 helps you do that. The next step is getting regular exercise. Exercise goes hand in hand with diet changes, and it's crucial for improved health and well-being. Exercise helps you

✔ **Battle depression.** Depression is a major hypoglycemia symptom that endorphins, which are released with you're active, can work to fight. (See Chapter 4 for more on endorphins.)

✔ **Gain insulin sensitivity.** Increased sensitivity results in lower blood insulin levels. (Chapter 2 gives you details about how hypoglycemia works.)

✔ **Boost self-confidence.** This boost includes better body image and more control over other aspects of life.

✔ **Achieve and maintain your ideal weight.** This is another critical issue for a hypoglycemic. (Chapter 6 tells you more about this.)

✔ **Stick to a healthy diet.** After you get into shape, your body will seem to pull you toward good carbs, protein, fruits, and vegetables.

✔ **Become stronger and healthier.** When you're strong and healthy, you don't need to be quite as compulsive about your diet. You can eat more carbs, and you can even eat forbidden foods on occasion without suffering undue consequences. Interested?

Keep these things in mind before getting started:

✔ Always see a doctor before participating in a fitness program. (Chapter 5 gives you doc-picking info.)

✔ Pick an activity that you're suited for and that appeals to you.

✔ Enjoy many activities. Do a variety of exercises to keep from getting bored. As a matter of fact, doing a variety is good because you work different parts of your body.

✔ If you already have an exercise routine but you're not getting the results you want, review it. Keeping track of your progress in your food journal (flip to Chapter 6) is a good way to start. Write down the type of activity, along with the intensity and duration.

If you want more general knowledge and comprehensive guidance on how to get fit, check out *Fitness For Dummies,* by Susanne Schlosberg and Liz Neporent (Wiley Publishing).

Timing Your Carbs

The subject of carbs is of vital importance to anyone who's struggling with erratic blood sugar levels. That's because carbohydrates most directly affect the sugar in your blood. (For a complete discussion on carbs and blood sugar, see Chapters 2 and 6.) The short version? When you begin exercising, hormones are released into the bloodstream signaling the liver and fat cells to liberate their stored energy nutrients, primarily glucose. How much *glycogen* (the sugar your body stores) you have in store depends partly on the amount of carbs in your diet.

When you exercise, your body uses up a lot of glucose, which needs replenishing. You need to know what to eat and when to prevent a blood sugar crash.

Studies have shown that eating carbs an hour before exercising can extend endurance and improve performance. If you're going to take part in a strenuous form of exercise for more than 90 minutes, such as mountain climbing, cross-country skiing, aerobics, or gym workouts, your best bet is to eat a meal containing carbs about one to two hours before the event. Doing so allows time for the food to leave the stomach and reach the small intestine. You don't want to eat too close to your workout; otherwise, food will still be in your stomach and you may get nauseated.

On the other hand, if you eat about two hours or more before your workout, most of the carbs will have already been burned up. The trick, therefore, is to eat something that's very slowly digested, so that it remains in the intestine hours after consumption. You want food that's packaged in such a way that it's slowly digested, absorbed, and gradually released from the intestine into the blood-stream.

What carbs should you choose? Select foods with a GI (glycemic index) of less than 55, including those listed in Chapter 6. The body needs carbohydrates as fuel, but eating foods with a high GI will spare you problems. After an intense workout, however, a high GI food can help to restore the glycogen in muscles in time for the next event. If you're not a particularly athletic person, and you don't reg-ularly participate in events, you don't need to worry so much about replenishing your glycogen store. If you're famished after exercise, eat something that will quickly restore your blood sugar, and follow that with a high-GI carbohydrate and a little bit of protein.

Improving Insulin and Feeling the Burn: Aerobics

Burn, baby, burn. Aerobics gives you the good kind of burn. *Aerobic* literally means "with air." And you need extra air for sure when you do aerobic exercise. Aerobic exercise is any activity that gets your heart pumping faster and your lungs taking in more oxygen. Walking, bicycling, swimming, stair climbing — and yes, sex — count as aerobic exercise.

Talking the talk and walking

You can walk the walk or talk the talk, but walking definitely improves your health faster than talking. Walking is a simple and easy activity that just about anybody can do, which makes it one of the best exercises for improving your health. Walking makes the body more sensitive to the effects of insulin and thus allows more glucose to be absorbed by the cells. Any exercise that improves insulin function is good for people who have problems metabolizing glucose or regulating blood sugar.

Walking has been proven to help people reduce their cravings for addictive substances, such as nicotine, alcohol, and barbiturates. If you're hypoglycemic, one of the worst things you can do is abuse a substance like liquor or tobacco, but when you're addicted, quitting is hard to do. Use walking as your tool for fighting those cravings and keeping your hypoglycemia under control.

Walking, an aerobic workout, is especially good for the blood-sugar challenged, because it's easy to get started and keep up (even if you're suffering from fatigue), and it doesn't have complex routines to memorize (if you're suffering from brain fog). If you're out of shape, or if you've been otherwise inactive for a long time, walking may be the best way for you to begin exercising. After you exercise with walking for a while, you can simply continue with it or use it as a transitional activity for other sports.

Bad air days

Did you know that a growing body of research suggests that exposure to natural light for one and a half to two hours a day may activate the adrenal glands and thereby support adrenal function? Because the adrenals are involved with normal blood sugar regulation, people with low blood sugar may do well to get some sun every day.

A really good way to get some sunlight is to exercise outdoors. Not only is it invigorating but it will also help your body acclimatize to the changing seasons better. Plus, working out in the mornings boosts your mood. Better overall health can also translate into better blood sugar regulation. But you need to watch out for bad air days:

- If there's a pollution alert, don't needlessly expose yourself.

- Don't jog in the smog.

- Apply sunscreen, with an SPF rating of at least 15, that blocks both UVA and UVB rays.

- Don't wear perfume in the sun, because some perfumes contain ingredients that can cause burns or rashes when exposed to sunlight. Besides, the mix of perfume and sweat isn't the most alluring scent.

- Wear a helmet if you're participating in an activity that requires one (such as biking), especially if you're prone to dizzy spells from attacks of low blood sugar.

Here are some walking do's and don'ts:

Do's

✔ Before a walk that will last an hour or more, eat a snack with some protein and a complex carb. This snack will ensure that you don't tire out from your blood sugar dropping mid-track.

✔ Carry a snack and a water bottle with you.

✔ Use exercise walking, which combines arm and leg movements. *Fitness Walking For Dummies,* by Liz Neporent (Wiley Publishing), informs you of every aspect of walking.

✔ Get the right shoes. Your shoes should be flexible, have breathable fabrics, and provide good traction. Look for cushioning at the tongue, around the collar, and at the heel. If you walk fast, look for cushioning at the ball of the foot, also.

✔ If you tend to get dizzy or easily exhausted, walk at night rather than in the morning.

✔ Get a weighted vest. They're specially designed for walking, and you can get one that allows you to increase the weight as you become better conditioned. The weights increase resistance and help you burn more calories. Most people can start out with very low weights in the vest, but if you're very much out of shape, don't wear a vest until you're in better shape.

Don'ts

✔ Don't walk while wearing ankle or wrist weights. You may injure yourself from the added strain. (Weighted vests apply the weight more evenly and are therefore less likely to cause problems.)

✔ Don't wear weights (vest or otherwise) that are more than 10 percent of your body weight. You may otherwise develop back problems.

✔ Don't forget to replace your walking shoes every 400 miles (or when they start showing wear).

What's the difference, you ask? Running and jogging

Running and jogging (a faster version of running) are good exercises, and they're darn good ways to get your blood circulating and burn up calories. However, if you have low blood pressure — as many hypoglycemics do — and if bouts of low blood sugar have left you more weary than not, it may be too much to suddenly start running. A good workout combination is running and walking. For instance, walk fast for 10 minutes, run for 1 minute, and then walk at a normal pace for another 10 minutes.

For maximum aerobic benefit, jog at least 20 minutes at your *target heart rate*. The target rate shows you how fast your heart should beat per minute when you exercise. To calculate your individual heart rate:

> Subtract your age from 226 if you're a woman, and 220 if you're a man.
>
> Multiply the result by .80. This is your maximum target heart rate.
>
> Multiply the result by .70. This is your minimum target heart rate.

For example, say I'm a 96-year-old man:

> $220 - 96 = 124$
>
> $124 \times .70 = 86.8$ (maximum target heart rate)
>
> $86.8 \times .80 = 69.44$ (minimum target heart rate)

Don't worry if you can't maintain your target heart rate for 20 minutes. Recent studies have shown that you can get similar benefits even with 5-minute workouts interspersed at various times of the day. And if you can't get outside to run, run in place; the intensity won't be the same, but anything is better than sitting on your butt.

As with most exercises that involve your feet, shoes are an extremely important part of running. The proper shoes ensure that you get the most out of your workout and avoid injury. You can read more about what to look for in shoes in this chapter's previous section, and you can also buy your running shoes from a store that specializes in runners' needs. With this type of store, you can use the knowledge of the experts to be sure that you're buying the best shoes for your feet.

Shaking your groove thang: Dancing

You don't need to boogie all night to get the benefits of dance. This fantastic activity can make you chipper, dapper, and slimmer — *and* it can lift you right up from the doldrums of the low blood sugar blues. And you're not limited to any one kind of dance. You can choose from all different types of dance: jazz, modern, hip hop,

African, belly, and folk, to name just a few. You can do it solo, in a pair, or as a group.

Whether you're married or a singleton, you can add a little oomph into your love life by dancing as a couple or getting your body revved up with dance. But what does this oomph have to do with low blood sugar? Plenty! When you're so often weary, down in the dumps, or crabby as a result of your hypoglycemia, love and lust can leach away and fizzle down to a most unfortunate finale. So if your hypoglycemic syndrome has put a strain in your relationship, what better way to put the sparkle back than through dance? (Chapters 13 and 14 address relationship issues at length.)

If you've been sidelined by hypoglycemia for a long time, don't overdo it. Make sure that you find a class that's appropriate to your fitness level. Ballroom dancing and folk dance are generally pretty safe, but make sure that you tell your instructor about any physical problems you have.

Regulating Blood Sugar with Yoga and T'ai Chi

Yoga and T'ai Chi (and related forms) are specifically designed to promote mental, emotional, and spiritual growth along with physical fitness. Although quite different in practice, T'ai Chi and yoga do have similarities. They're both comprehensive forms of exercise that work the entire body, tone and build muscles, strengthen the organs and musculoskeletal structure, and improve circulation of the *qi* (also spelled ch'i) — the life force that courses through the body.

Both T'ai Chi and yoga fit well into *comprehensive treatment* programs for diabetes and hypoglycemia that involve mind, body, and spirit. These ailments have a genetic component, but other contributing factors are diet, sedentary habits, and physical, emotional, and mental stress. All these factors are addressed in a holistic manner in the practices of T'ai Chi and yoga. (Chapter 5 talks more about holistic and Eastern approaches, as well.)

So which should you study? It depends on what you like, what feels most comfortable to you, and the instructors you can find.

Going yoga

Yoga, which started in India, consists of poses you hold from a few seconds to several minutes. Many forms, such as Hatha yoga and

Iyengar yoga, exist. Most forms include the same fundamental poses, but some classes focus more on sweating, some on breathing, and some on spirituality.

Numerous studies have reported the beneficial effect of the practice of yoga on regulating blood sugar control. Some even venture to claim that some cases of type 1 diabetes (what used to be known as *juvenile diabetes*) were controlled through the practice of yoga. (Chapter 2 has more info on diabetes.) The direct stimulation of the pancreas by certain yogic postures seems to stimulate and rejuvenate the pancreatic cells, which are responsible for producing insulin. Although the studies only dealt with the effect on diabetes, the findings suggest by implication that yoga is beneficial for hypoglycemia.

Taking T'ai Chi

T'ai Chi Chuan (also spelled "Taiji") has often been described as Chinese yoga. Because T'ai Chi is a set of smooth, flowing exercises, people tend to forget that it's a martial art. Although T'ai Chi actively discourages violence, you can learn fighting skills, such as sparring and self-defense. T'ai Chi is a *soft,* or internal, form of martial arts (as opposed to the *hard* external schools, such as Shaolin, karate, or Tae Kwon Do). Unlike the hard schools of martial arts, T'ai Chi is accessible to elderly or frail people, but it can also be rigorous and demanding.

Unless you already have a background in martial arts, don't attempt to learn T'ai Chi from a video. Unlike aerobics or dance, learning T'ai Chi properly without the physical presence of a qualified instructor is extremely difficult, if not impossible. If you try to learn T'ai Chi without an instructor, you'll likely pick up bad habits that will be hard to correct later on. Do yourself a favor and find a class and instructor that you really like.

Although hydration is important when exercising, you shouldn't drink liquids for at least 15 minutes before practicing T'ai Chi. You should also avoid eating 30 minutes before and after practice. Unless you're extremely dehydrated, avoid drinking water (especially if the water's cold) during the practice. Drinking liquids can cool your body too much and put a damper on the really good flow of qi that your workout sets in motion.

Kicking Weakness with Weights

You don't need to become a muscle-bound lifter to benefit from weight training. Building more muscle is one of the most effective ways to boost your metabolism, lose weight, tone up, and build bone density (which can help stave off osteoporosis).

It's very important to have a *spotter* (someone to help you lift the dumbbell on and off the rack) when you're working with weights. Spotters can help you if you have trouble completing a set and keep you from getting hurt. And don't be too cavalier when handling dumbbells and other weights.

In addition to helping spot you, a personal trainer or qualified person from your gym can ensure that you're getting the proper workout and that you're correctly using the weights. Make sure that you learn how to lift weights correctly before lifting them solo at home, unless you're only using 1- to 5-pound dumbbells. Even then, proper training is important.

Clearing Brain Fog with Qigong

Brain fog is mental confusion, a feeling that often accompanies hypoglycemia. (For more on brain fog, see Chapter 3.) And what is *qigong?* Simply put, it's a Chinese system of physical training, philosophy, and comprehensive preventive and therapeutic health-care that involves breathing exercises and meditation. It's somewhat related to T'ai Chi and other soft forms of martial arts, but it doesn't have any of the hard elements of martial arts, such as kicks and strikes.

The *qi* in qigong refers to breath, vital essence, and life force; *gong* means skill, work, and self-discipline. Many scientific studies have been done on the numerous benefits of qigong. Most importantly for hypoglycemics, qigong has been found to help regulate blood sugar by strengthening the *endocrine system,* blood sugar's regulator.

How would you like to wash your brain, cleanse your marrow, and change your muscles and tendons? Before you say, "No thanks!" rest assured that it's not as gory as it sounds. Qigong involves no blood or surgery. We're actually referring to the titles of the classic qigong moves — Xi Sui Jing (or Marrow/Brain Washing Classic) and Yi Jin Jing (or Muscle/Tendon Changing Classic). They were written by a famous Chinese physician, Bian Que, and they describe a form of qigong that uses breathing to increase qi circulation.

These ancient classics give prescriptions for using qigong to gain, attain, and maintain vibrant health, helping to change the body from weak to strong, strengthen the blood and immune system, and energize the brain. If you do it right, you'll be better able to sense your body, which can help you tune in more to the diet your body actually needs, rather than to what an outside authority or some school of thought tells you.

There are more than 3,000 varieties of qigong. Proper instruction is important (just like T'ai Chi, you can't really learn qigong through a book or a video, although you can use those tools as supplements), and so is regular practice. You need to have patience, persistence, and commitment to enjoy the full benefits of qigong. Give qigong a minimum of three months and up to a year before expecting to see any changes. Oh, and one more thing: Avoid sexual intercourse for at least one hour before and after a qigong session. Having sex an hour before or after a session may interfere with your training because it can impede flow of qi.

Mastering the martials

Studying the fighting arts for your health is something you may want to consider. Through the practice, you'll cultivate discipline, commitment, self-confidence, strength, and directness of purpose — the diametric opposite of how you are when weak and debilitated by your system's metabolic glitch. It'll definitely clear any cobwebs in your brain and make your thinking sharp. You'll hardly remember what brain fog was like.

✔ Do a little research to find out which martial arts may appeal to you most.

✔ Make sure that you find a true master of the arts.

✔ Beware of anyone who claims that his particular style of martial arts is the one and only, who claims to know all the answers, or who demands an inordinate amount of your time and/or money. If anyone starts asking for your first born, it's a sure sign that you should bail out!

Strictly from a health standpoint, the soft, or internal, school of martial arts (like T'ai Chi) is generally considered more effective. The internal school of martial arts emphasizes the cultivation of qi (instead of brute force) and teaches you how to use your opponent's strength against him.

Then there's kickboxing, which has found adherents among women, and Tae Bo, which incorporates moves from martial arts for an aerobic workout — so it's not exactly a martial art per se. (Kickboxing and Tae Bo are considered hard forms.) Then, of course, you have your traditional martial arts from China, Japan, Korea, and other countries. Aside from T'ai Chi, other internal schools of martial arts include Hsing Yi and Bagua Zhang.

Part IV
Emulating Lifestyles of the Well and Healthy

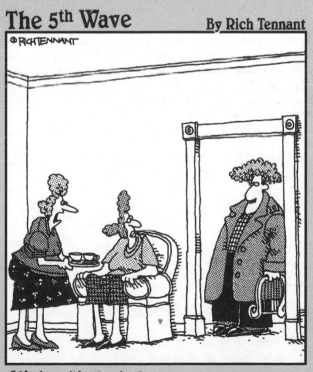

The 5th Wave   By Rich Tennant

"Oh dear, it's Troy's Harpo—glycemia. I can always tell — fatigue, confusion, the compulsion to play the harp in a trench coat and fright—wig..."

In this part . . .

In this section, we help you map out a lifestyle for achieving the vibrant health you desire. You chart a course through the two indispensable pillars for building a solid foundation for health: diet and exercise. They don't have to be complicated, difficult, or unpleasant. Quite the contrary. You should find yourself appreciating your new lifestyle. We show you how to create a practical and doable diet. You explore the wonderful world of movement, and you figure out how to choose exercises that are fun for you. When it comes to revving your body up, there's nothing like exercise. Now it's time to get rolling.

Chapter 9

All Stressed Out and Nowhere to Go

*H*ave you been swinging high, swinging low, singing the blood sugar blues? Stress will do that to you.

Stress can hinder attempts to balance your blood sugar level. When you're stressed, a series of biochemical changes take place to prepare you to deal with your stressors: the old *fight-or-flight response*. When primitive man saw a saber-toothed tiger, he needed a burst of energy to fight or flee from the predator. Unless you're a big game hunter, you don't often run into hungry tigers or lions. (Only kitty cats pestering you for food.) Today, we're more likely to encounter threats in the form of job layoffs or work deadlines. But just like in the good ol' days of yore, the adrenal glands continue to pump you full of adrenaline so that you can either hightail it out of there or do battle. When you deal with stress day after day, your body begins to break down.

To compound the problem, many people turn to food when they're faced with continued stress. We sure don't need to tell you that most people aren't grabbing a celery stick or a bowl of steamed green beans to help themselves deal with stress. Most people use sugar as a quick pick-me-up. In response to the sugar, the body secretes too much insulin, as well as — guess what — more adrenaline! And the vicious cycle is perpetuated. This cycle is even more vicious if you happen to be hypoglycemic, because of the problem you already have with balancing your blood sugar.

Ah, but don't get stressed-out over stress. Knowing how to handle stress will in turn help you handle your hypoglycemia. This chapter is here to rescue you.

Knotting Off

Because stress can have an adverse effect on your body, figuring out how to handle and get rid of it is critical. The art of relaxation — and it truly is an art — is the key to healthy living. If you have a health condition, you better listen up! You can alleviate many hypoglycemic symptoms with proper relaxation techniques. If you are sugar-balance-challenged, you will find these techniques indispensable as you transition to a healthier diet. Making healthy changes doesn't have to be a grin-and-bear-it situation. If you use the methods outlined here and take the vitamins that help to curb any food cravings (see Chapter 7 for supplements and other natural remedies), you'll be able to make a smooth transition to a healthy lifestyle.

You need to keep in mind that, while you may start noticing improvements almost immediately, it may be weeks or months before you're free of the physical and emotional problems associated with hypoglycemia. However, you can gain immediate relief by the progressive relaxation of your muscles. The relaxation exercises help with anxiety, depression, and fatigue, among other things, and unlike medication, they don't cause any negative side effects.

Don't stress this test

Take the Holmes-Rahe Social Adjustment Rating Scale test to help determine how stressed out you are: http://www.bcbsaz.com/connect/fyhealth/vitality543.asp. This stress test is valid whether you have blood sugar imbalances or not. You'll notice that each life event has a number assigned to it, from a low of 10 to a high of 100.

So how did you do? Anything below 100 means you may be stressed out from boredom. (Just kidding, of course. But if you do want to jazz up your life, try salsa dancing.) As a character in a famous Chinese cartoon Lao Fu Tze quipped, "Yours is the case of hypertension caused by over-relaxation." (However, if you are the type of person who gets easily stressed, even a score of 150 can indicate high stress.)

Before you can learn how to relax your muscles, you need to recognize when they're tense. You can recognize the tension by consciously tuning in to your body. If you're one of those people who live primarily in their heads, you're more likely to lend your ears to telemarketers than to your own body. Now you have a chance to get in touch with how your body feels.

 The following progressive muscle relaxation exercise helps you feel the difference between relaxed and tense muscles. It also helps you discover how to loosen up those tightly wound muscles. When performing this exercise, avoid overstraining yourself.

1. **Go somewhere quiet where you won't be disturbed.**

2. **Lie down on a bed (or wherever you can get comfortable).**

3. **Loosen any clothes that may be too tight.**

4. **Take a few breaths in and out.**

5. **Place your hand on your stomach and breathe in deeply while you press down.**

    Feel how your stomach expands when you breathe deeply.

6. **Tense your feet and curl your toes downward.**

    Hold for a few seconds and then release.

    Don't hold your breath. Breathe normally for the rest of the exercise.

7. **Tense your calves so that your toes are bent towards your face.**

    Don't tighten so much that you get cramps. Hold for a few seconds and then relax.

8. **Tighten your sphincter muscles (in the anal region).**

    Hold and release.

9. **Tighten your buttocks and thighs.**

    Hold and release. Feel the difference between tight and relaxed muscles.

10. **Clench your fists as you also tighten your forearms and upper arms.**

    Hold for a few seconds and then release.

11. **Shrug your shoulders and bring them up toward your ears.**

    Hold and release.

12. **Tighten your stomach.**

    Hold and release.

13. **Arch your back without straining.**

    Hold and release. Be very careful if you have a back problem.

14. **Open your mouth wide and feel the tension in your jaw and neck.**

    Be careful not to tense up too much, as you may hurt yourself. Hold for a few seconds and then relax. Your lips should be slightly parted.

15. **Squeeze your eyes closed tight and then relax.**

    Keep your eyes closed and feel the warmth spread across your eyelids.

16. **Raise your eyebrows as high as they will go so that your forehead gets wrinkled.**

    Hold and release. Smooth out your forehead completely.

17. **Tense your entire body.**

    Hold for several seconds and then release. Repeat this step two more times. When you're finished, you should feel a pleasant wave of relaxation sweep over you. All of your muscles will feel loose and soft. Try to remember this sensation.

With this exercise, you feel how the sensations of tension and relaxation differ. It lets you know how you're supposed to feel when you're relaxed. As you keep practicing, it becomes easier for you to induce this state of relaxation. For instance, assume that you agreed to go out to eat with your friends even though you feel somewhat volatile. Then, someone suggests chipping in on a meal that's definitely off-limits for you. You don't want the situation to stress you out. You need to be able to take care of yourself without antagonizing anyone. What should you do? At times like this, you can do a mini-version of the muscle relaxation technique by tensing the muscles of your arms and legs and then releasing them. This shortened version will help diffuse any tension you may feel.

Breathing Helps Your Blood Sugar

Do you want a quick, fast stress fix? Something that will deliver an instant boost, get you turbocharged, and make you tingle with life and energy? Okay, then take a deep breath. And then another. There you have it: Breathing is the elixir of life. Breathing is something you can do at any time. And it costs absolutely nothing. It helps you become less irritated, less depressed, and less prone to such problems as panic attacks, anxiety, muscle tension, headaches, and fatigue (all of which are symptoms of hypoglycemia). That's right, deep breathing can help you alleviate many distressing symptoms. It can also help you beat food addictions and food cravings.

People have attested to giving up all kinds of addictions, such as cigarette smoking and candy bars, just by deep breathing. Despite all the benefits gained from deep breathing, most people are under-breathers who are totally stingy about the way they breathe. (You'd think that they were being charged by the minute or the gallon.) Unless you're the exception, you probably suffer from a lack of serious breathing (especially if you have any health issues, including hypoglycemia).

So guess what our message is? If you said that it's about how deep breathing helps balance your blood sugar (by helping the organs of your body to function more efficiently), you're one smart cookie. (And please, if you're getting a craving for cookies, just hold off. For tips on beating temptations, see the Cheat Sheet at the front of the book.)

In addition to your regular deep-breathing sessions, you should switch to your deep-breathing mode when you feel

- ✔ Dizzy
- ✔ Lightheaded
- ✔ Irritated
- ✔ Angry
- ✔ Anxious
- ✔ Fatigued
- ✔ Achy
- ✔ Cravings for sugar or simple starches (cakes, croissants, colas, fries, and so on)

Here's a very basic breathing technique that everyone should try. This technique is a handy-dandy way to perk you up anytime you're feeling dragged out. It can be a good way to start out the morning. Come to think of it, you may want to use it to end the day, too.

1. **Inhale through your nose for a count of four to six (as many you can manage comfortably).**

2. **Hold the air in your lungs for a count of four to six.**

Hold for the same number of counts as your inhalation. In other words, if you inhaled for a count of four, hold for a count of four.

3. Exhale through your nose for a count of four to six.

If you inhaled for a count of four, exhale for a count of four.

You can practice this technique when you have a bit of time to yourself:

1. Lie down on a rug or exercise mat on the floor and bend your knees, keeping your feet about shoulder width apart.

2. Relax any areas of your body that are tight.

If you like, do the progressive muscle relaxation technique described earlier in this chapter.

3. Keep your mouth closed but relaxed.

4. Put one hand on your chest and the other on your stomach.

5. Breathe in deeply through your nose to the count of five.

Your abdomen should push up into your hand as much as possible. Your chest, however, should move only slightly. The hand on your chest will allow you to determine if you are moving your chest too much.

6. Exhale through your mouth.

7. Continue deep breathing for 5 to 20 minutes.

The great thing about these breathing exercises is that they make you feel instantly revived. You'll get the most benefit, though, if you make these exercises a regular practice. After several months of these breathing exercises, you may even be able to blow down a brick house (although I wouldn't hold my breath waiting for that to happen). At the very least, your friends will be impressed by the dynamo that you've become. Just don't try deep breathing on the phone.

Surfing the Alpha Wave with Meditation

Meditation occurs when you become relaxed and aware and have a heightened sense of alertness. This effective antidote for stress and tension induces mental tranquility and physical relaxation, reduces high blood pressure, and improves circulation. Because hypoglycemia can be a stressor in itself, this is definitely good news for hypoglycemics. Studies also show that meditating can boost the intensity of *alpha waves,* brain waves associated with quiet, receptive states of the mind that are conducive to relaxation and creativity.

For all you hyper-driven go-getters, rest assured that meditating isn't the same as vegetating. Nor does meditating have to be anything quaint or mystical — you don't have to sprout a beard and sit in the lotus position in front of a temple. Think of meditation as a way of focusing your mind on one thing. If you're confused, distracted, or anxious — all side effects of low blood sugar — meditation can help you to not only concentrate but to achieve serenity. Countless studies have shown the benefit of regular meditation in relieving stress and promoting good health. Meditation helps alleviate high blood pressure, heart disease, diabetes, arthritis, anxiety, depression, and so on. It can definitely aid you in regulating your blood sugar and anything else that's off kilter.

Balancing your blood and body

Some doctors suspect that the symptoms of hypoglycemia may be caused more by the release of stress hormones than by low blood sugar. If this theory is true, hypoglycemics should be able to drastically reduce the frequency and severity of their symptoms through the practice of meditation. It's been scientifically proven that meditating on a regular basis can relieve chronic pain, lower levels of stress hormones, and improve circulation. Just what the doctor ordered.

A smorgasbord of meditations is out there for you to choose from. You can try Zen meditation, transcendental meditation, Tibetan Buddhist meditations, Taoist meditation, and insight meditation (also called Vipassana), to name just a few. Check out *Meditation For Dummies,* by Stephan Bodian (Wiley Publishing), for further information.

Here's a simple meditation using a *mantra* (a type of incantation or affirmation):

1. **Sit in a chair or on the floor.**

   Sit wherever is most comfortable for you. Keep your back straight.

2. **Close your eyes, take a few deep breaths, relax, and try to quiet your mind.**

3. **Repeat the word *om* silently to yourself.**

   Or make up a hypo-specific mantra, such as "I'm becoming healthier."

   Don't worry if you keep having distracting thoughts. Just bring your awareness back to the mantra and continue repeating it. Try it for anywhere from 5 to 20 minutes.

4. **Take a few deep breaths and slowly open your eyes.**

You may be aware of a lot of thoughts during this meditation. You may even forget that you're supposed to be meditating. (Don't worry if you do; most people have that experience.) Through regular meditation practice, you can discover how to train the *monkey mind,* that unruly, undisciplined mind that flits from one thought to the next. When your mind chatter is turned down to a reasonable volume, you may find your mind becoming serene — more like the surface of a quiet lake rather than a turbulent stream.

 To start off, meditate for just five minutes a day. If you make meditation a habit, you'll be able to gradually go longer. Experienced practitioners meditate for an hour or even longer. Meditate for the amount of time that fits your schedule, but do make meditation a regular practice. The important thing is to meditate every day. As with anything, practice, patience, and persistence are what count the most.

If you don't like repeating words, you may want to try another basic meditation where you pay attention to your breathing. This meditation is great for toning the belly and helping relieve constipation. It's also a great way to relax yourself before a test or an interview. Here's a variation from a Taoist form of meditation:

1. **Sit in a chair or cross-legged on the floor.**

   Keep your back straight and your shoulders relaxed and sloping downward. Avoid jutting out your chin: It should be tucked in slightly, but not too much.

2. **Relax your jaw and lightly touch your tongue on the inside of your upper front teeth.**

3. **Close your eyes partially so that you're gazing softly downward, not focusing on anything.**

4. **Bring your attention to your *Dan Tien,* which is located inside your abdomen about an inch below your belly button.**

   Think of the Dan Tien as your energy center, the cauldron in your belly. Dan Tien is the reservoir for your *qi,* or life force.

You can read more about Dan Tien in *T'ai Chi For Dummies,* by Therese Iknoian (Wiley Publishing). There are other locations for the Dan Tien, but this spot suits our purposes.

5. **Inhale deeply as you expand your abdomen.**

6. **Exhale as you contract your abdomen.**

   Keep your attention lightly centered on the Dan Tien as you inhale and exhale.

Aside from your regular sessions, you can meditate whenever you experience any pain or discomfort from the side effects of low blood sugar. Meditation can help enormously as you change to healthier eating habits. It can help lessen your mood swings; the contrast between the hills and valleys that you experience won't be quite so sharp. If you find yourself going up and down emotionally, try meditation, breathing exercises, or progressive muscle relaxation. Or combine all three!

Kicking food cravings in the gut

Because stress can trigger cravings for all the wrong foods — sugar, sugar, and more sugar! — meditation, which alleviates stress, can be especially beneficial.

As you develop a mindfulness with meditation, you become more aware of your eating habits. As much as people may be obsessed with food, most don't pay sufficient attention to what they're eating. In fact, many people seem to go almost unconscious when they eat.

To become more conscious about your eating, try the following meditation:

1. **Pick a time when you're home alone.**

   If you live with people, do the meditation in your room or someplace where you can have privacy, and ask everyone not to disturb you.

2. **Place the food in front of you.**

   This can be any food (good, bad, or indifferent) that you're about to eat. The object is to become more aware of what you're eating.

3. **Take several deep breaths.**

4. **Note the color, shape, and texture of the food.**

   - **Note any reactions you have.** How do you feel about the food? Does it look appealing to you?

   - **Notice how your body reacts to the food.** What physical sensations do you have?

5. **Now bring the food to your mouth.**

   - **Smell the food.** What is your reaction to the smell?

   - **Take a bite.** How does it feel to bite into the food?

   - **Chew the food.** How does the food feel to your lips, teeth, and tongue? What other sensations do you notice?

   - **As you swallow the food, pay attention to how your esophagus contracts and relaxes.** Can you feel the food traveling down to your stomach?

   - **Note how your stomach feels after you swallow the food.**

6. **Put the food down between bites and breathe deeply.**

7. **Take another bite.**

   Again, pay attention to all the sensations.

This meditation helps you become more conscious of the act of eating. You can also try this meditation when you're eating a forbidden food. Rather than cram your food down in a rush or with a feeling of guilt, be as fully conscious as you can when you eat. And enjoy what you're eating! If paying attention to all the details gets tedious after awhile, just remain focused on the taste and smell of the food, and relish it as much as you can.

Making the Ultimate Smoothie: Hypno-Soothing

Self-hypnosis is another tool you can use if you hit rough patches in your effort to transition to a hypoglycemic diet. You can use it to help stick to your food plan or alleviate uncomfortable hypoglycemic symptoms. (For more tips on tackling temptations, see the Cheat Sheet at the front of the book.)

Don't be spooked by the word *hypnosis*. It's not witchcraft, and it's not a séance. And you won't be clucking around like a hen either, because self-hypnosis is not the same as stage hypnosis, where the focus is on showmanship rather than healing. You should find it very relaxing, in fact. With self-hypnosis, you're the one in charge. You maintain total control. It's not dangerous, and you can do it alone.

You can hypnotize yourself in many different ways. Here's one simple method:

1. **Pick a quiet time and place where you won't be disturbed.**

2. **Play soothing music if you think that it may help you, especially if background noise is a problem.**

3. **Lie down where you can be comfortable.**

   If you find that you keep falling asleep when you try to hypnotize yourself, sit in a chair.

4. **Inhale slowly and deeply.**

   Hold your breath and exhale slowly. Each time you exhale, imagine that you're releasing all your tension.

5. **Use the progressive muscle relaxation technique described earlier in this chapter to help release all your tensions.**

   Work from your toes up, relaxing each muscle group.

6. **If your neck is stiff, do a few slow head rolls and really work to get your muscles relaxed.**

7. **Take as much time as you need to get fully relaxed.**

   It will take longer in the beginning, but later you'll achieve relaxation quickly.

8. **Imagine that you're in an elevator.**

   The floor indicator shows that you are on the 50th floor. The elevator begins to go down at a steady pace, not too fast, not too slow. You're on the 49th floor, and you're going down, down, down. Continue breathing deeply and slowly as you watch the numbers go down . . . 48th, 47th, and so on.

   If thoughts or other images intrude, just gently brush them aside.

   With each breath, you're going deeper and deeper.

9. **When the elevator arrives at the first floor, you're ready to give yourself suggestions.**

10. **You should now give yourself autosuggestions.**

    Autosuggestions are statements that you repeat while in a hypnotic state to influence your own attitudes and behavior. Use words and statements that make sense to you, as they will be more effective.

For example, you can say, "I naturally gravitate toward healthy foods," or "I'm finding it easier and easier to eat a healthy diet with plenty of fresh vegetables and fruits," or "I can now easily pass up processed foods that are filled with sugar and starch."

You can also make up statements to help ease your symptoms, such as, "I am now happy and emotionally balanced, and I'm becoming more and more energetic each day."

Make all your statements affirmative and in the present tense. Don't say, "I will not eat dessert anymore." Instead try, "I no longer have a desire for desserts that are full of sugar."

After you make your suggestion, you're ready to terminate the session.

11. **Terminate your session by counting to three.**

Say, "I'm going to count from one to three. At the count of three, I'll be totally refreshed, wide awake, and completely alert. One — I'm beginning to come out of it. Two — I'm coming out more, ready to wake up. Three — I'm wide awake, feeling refreshed and revitalized."

As with anything, you need to set up a regular time of practice, and you need to do it consistently, or you won't get the results you want. You won't get instant results, but you should start to see some changes in a few weeks. If you don't notice changes during this time, examine your suggestions and try different ones. If you feel you need more support and advice on what to do, consider trying one of the numerous books and tapes on self-hypnosis. However, the information outlined here should be enough to get you going.

Chapter 10

Defanging the Depression Demons

Watch out for the demons of depression. If you have chronic problems with low blood sugar, they're sure to attack you sooner or later. Of course, they're not real demons with horns and fangs. In a way, though, these demons are much more frightening, because they're invisible and they attack one of your most vulnerable areas — your state of mind.

Why is depression one of hypoglycemia's main symptoms? Because its sisters — anxiety, irritability, poor concentration, feelings of panic, and suicidal tendencies — are just a few things hypoglycemia can create. Hypoglycemics also tend to suffer from temper tantrums, mood swings, and crying jags. (See Chapter 3 for more symptom info.) These symptoms aren't surprising, considering that the brain uses glucose as its fuel. When there isn't enough glucose circulating in your blood, your brain begins to starve. At rest, the brain consumes ⅓ of the body's total glucose requirement.

This chapter sheds light on how to deal with stresses that may be keeping you hooked to the hypoglycemic cycle of eating the wrong foods, making you feel even sicker and causing you to reach for foods that trigger bouts of hypoglycemia . . . and on and on.

Revealing another Epidemic

According to the National Institute of Mental Health (NIMH), an estimated 6.7 million people in established market economies, such as the United States, suffer from depression. That's 6.8 percent of the population. In fact, major depression (not just your ordinary everyday blues, but a serious medical condition) is the leading cause of disability worldwide. These statistics may seem misleading, because many people are unaware of their depression while others resist seeking proper treatment. Depression still tends to be regarded as a character defect or a weakness of will rather than as a multifaceted illness.

Not only is depression the most undertreated medical illness, it's also the most treatable. Treatment is said to be effective in more than 80 percent of cases. Perhaps most of the cases that have been resistant to treatment can be affected through proper dietary changes.

To help you recognize the symptoms of depression in yourself and others, here are some questions adapted from the National Institutes of Health:

- Are you persistently sad?
- Do you feel "empty" most of the time, and do you feel that life is meaningless?
- Has your energy decreased lately? Do you feel tired most of the time?
- Do you no longer find pleasure in activities you used to enjoy, including sex?
- Have you been experiencing sleep disturbances? Is it hard for you to sleep? Do you wake up in the middle of the night or early in the morning? Do you oversleep?
- Have you recently lost or gained a lot of weight? Have you lost your appetite? Do you overeat?
- Do you suffer from feelings of guilt, worthlessness, or helplessness?
- Have you been feeling more irritable than usual?
- Do you cry frequently?
- Do you have chronic aches and pains that don't respond to medical treatment?
- Do you have thoughts of death or suicide? Have you made any suicide attempts?

But how does sugar make you feel?

People often show affection and reward others by offering sugary treats. In most Western cultures (and other cultures, as well), sugar has become its own reward system. People have become conditioned to crave gooey desserts. As a result, so many emotional issues (not to mention excess weight) revolve around excess sugar consumption.

Sugar, therefore, can become a compulsive habit. For some, it becomes a true addiction. (To read more about sugar and addiction, flip to Chapter 3.) You know if you're an addict. Your friends may be able to eat a few cookies and leave the rest; get a few scoops of ice cream without devouring the entire tub; or eat just one square of a chocolate bar. But you? If you're a sugar junkie, you know what you do. And it's not pretty. If you're addicted to sugar, you may need to completely abstain from the substance, at least temporarily, to free yourself from your addiction. No matter what's causing your craving for sugar, you may be able to meet it by eating fruits or an occasional natural dessert made without refined sugar.

If you answer yes to the last question, immediately call 911, a suicide prevention hotline (whose number should be in the yellow pages), or your company's confidential employee assistance program. You also need to call if you think that someone else is considering suicide.

In addition, you may have difficulty remembering, concentrating, or making decisions. You may engage in destructive self-criticism or experience low self-esteem, and you may abuse drugs or alcohol. Bear in mind that these are all hallmarks of low blood sugar. Many unwitting sufferers become *substance addicts* in an unconscious effort to medicate themselves.

If you've had five or more of these symptoms for two weeks or longer, you may be suffering from depression. You owe it to yourself to seek professional help.

Knowing What (Gray) Matters

The brain is that gray matter we so-matter-of-factly take for granted. Brain cells, or *neurons,* communicate by releasing a chemical called a *neurotransmitter.* To put it simply, our moods change in response to the fluctuating levels of these neurotransmitters.

A deficiency or imbalance in any of these transmitters can cause problems such as depression, sleeplessness, and irritability. It's believed that a deficiency or imbalance of these neurotransmitters is the underlying cause of depression. As you can see from Table 10-1, many neurotransmitters perform various functions.

Table 10-1   Some Neurotransmitters and Their Functions

Major Neurotransmitters	Some of Their Functions
Endorphins	Elevate mood; act as a natural pain killer; produce loving feelings
Norepinephrine	Improves alertness; produces feelings of excitement and happiness; appetite control
Dopamine	Produces feelings of pleasure and euphoria; appetite control
Acetylcholine	Improves alertness, memory, and sexual performance
Phenylethylmine	Produces feelings of bliss and infatuation (Chocolate is a lover's delight because of its high levels of phenylethylmine!)
Serotonin	Relieves depression; diminishes cravings; improves self-confidence and impulse control

Getting Comfy on the Couch

Are you troubled, stressed, or depressed? If so, you may benefit from *psychotherapy* — therapy of the mind and emotions. *Psychotherapists,* professionals who administer psychotherapy, can help you find healthier ways to relate to others and unlearn behavior that leads to unwanted consequences.

So if you want to tackle bad habits that stem from hypoglycemia's physical causes (such as sugar addiction), or if just want to get yourself out of that funky depression (such as the one making you cry every other day), therapy may benefit you. To pick a good therapist, refer to Chapter 5; the suggestions for hooking up with the right doctor apply to therapists, as well.

Would you like some yin with your coffee?

From the point of view of traditional Chinese medicine, the desire for sweet flavor is seen as a craving for comfort and security, and a longing for the mother, which is a *yin* energy. Yin represents anything dark, female, cold, the earth, and so on. Its opposite, *Yang,* is regarded as male, light, warm, and heaven. The stressful urban setting is seen as having a yang energy, and city dwellers may unconsciously seek to balance the excessive yang by turning to sweets and starches, which are yin.

If your depression is mainly a result of blood sugar imbalance, you may find that no amount of talk therapy can keep the beast at bay until the underlying disorder is corrected. So don't use therapy as an excuse to shirk your diet. A healthy diet and therapy work hand-in-hand.

Therapy can help you deal better with hypoglycemic symptoms and tolerate the physical aches that are hypoglycemia's hallmark. At the same time, therapy can teach you to become more consistent at treating the disorder (for instance, by eating better and learning to incorporate exercise into your life). Ups and downs are inevitable while you're transitioning to a healthier lifestyle, and the support of a good therapist can be indispensable. *Psychology For Dummies,* by Adam Cash, PsyD (Wiley Publishing), discusses the various types of therapy and takes on tough therapy topics. Read it for more in-depth information.

Even if you choose not to see a therapist today, a plethora of self-help techniques can help you deal with mood disorders. Meditation, relaxation and progressive techniques, stress-management, and self-hypnosis mean that you'll never be bored. See Chapter 9 for more information about these subjects.

Learning new thinking skills

After years of suffering from low blood sugar, you or your loved one probably fell into the habit of distorted, negative thinking. You may worry too much, anticipate the worst, discount your achievements, get offended easily, and so on. You may feel as though you have no control over your feelings.

The good news is that anyone can learn how to replace damaging thoughts with more positive and realistic thoughts. When you tackle these counterproductive thoughts, it becomes easier to choose a lifestyle that supports your goals of maximum health and happiness.

Therapists teach you new ways of thinking and of looking at things by questioning your assumptions and pointing out the thoughts that lead to feelings of anxiety, depression, or other negatives. Therapy can help you regain control over your feelings by teaching you how to define and set goals, and how to take small, incremental steps toward achieving them. After you discover how to break your goals into small steps, you'll find it easier to make steady progress.

Books on changing your *cognitive patterns* can also be very helpful. Negative patterns of thinking feed depression. For instance, if you persistently think, "I'm a failure. There's nothing I can do to help myself," you're bound to feel helpless and hopeless. When you change these negative, habitual ways of thinking, you lift your mood. This is a useful therapy to try if you've been living with hypoglycemia and all its distorted thinking. Check out your local library or bookstore for good titles on the subject. Get books that guide you through changing your negative thoughts step-by-step and provide concrete examples.

Does he wear a whistle?

One alternative to therapy is to hire a life coach. A *life coach* acts like a personal trainer for your life. Athletes have coaches who train, motivate, and help them perform, so why shouldn't you have a coach to assist you in designing and creating a better life. Life coaches can help you set goals, teach you necessary skills, and keep you on track. Consultations are available in person, by phone, or by e-mail. Just as with therapists, you need to carefully screen potential coaches. Because life coaches are not required to undergo as rigorous a training program as psychotherapists, you need to be extra careful that you are hiring a person of integrity who can effectively guide you. Personal recommendations are probably the best.

Bear in mind that although coaches are supposed to honor confidentiality, they have no medical training, and they can't prescribe meds. Like sports coaches, they're good at motivating clients, but if you're currently suffering from depression, they'll be the first ones to tell you to see a licensed psychotherapist.

Thinking healthy

According to a controlled study by the University of Pennsylvania, people who maintain optimistic attitudes not only avoid depression but also improve their physical health. When students were taught *cognitive coping skills,* they reported fewer physical problems. In other words, they replaced self-defeating thoughts ("I'm too stupid to get good grades") with more positive ones ("I'm intelligent and can get good grades if I apply myself").

Similar coping skills can be applied to hypoglycemia. For instance, you may find yourself thinking, "How come everyone else gets to have fun eating whatever, while I have to restrict my diet. And I'm not even noticing any improvement." Not only are these thoughts negative, they're generally not even true. Replace these with more positive and more realistic thoughts. "If it's fun I want, there's lots I can do. Besides, I'm getting fewer headaches and my mood swings aren't as severe. Even though I miss my favorite foods, becoming healthier is worth giving up bad habits." From this example, you can see how easily you can discourage — or encourage — yourself.

Easing through the transition

When you've tackled counterproductive thoughts, it's easier to choose a lifestyle that supports your goals. A faulty body chemistry makes it difficult to make rational choices. If your battle with blood sugar imbalance has left you tired and weary, you can regain control by learning how to define and set goals and take small, incremental steps towards achieving them. If you don't know how to do this, read a book, take a course in goal-setting, or find a therapist who can help you define your goals.

Transitions can be difficult. One big plus about going on a recovery program for low blood sugar is that you start feeling so much better, and hence you're motivated to keep going. Of course, you may have setbacks and *plateaus* (when things stay the same and nothing seems to be happening), but if you honestly follow the food and exercise program, your symptoms will start disappearing, and you'll feel healthier.

This is where competent therapists can play a vital role. They teach you cognitive skills that you can use to address your transition. Also, you'll regain a sense of optimism knowing that you're tackling your problem head-on with a compassionate professional on your side.

Feeling Pro-Antidepressants

The hypoglycemic diet is your first and best line of offense for low blood sugar. (Chapter 6 starts you on that journey.) Exercise, discussed in Chapter 8, is your next best bet. Following that, your mental health is the place to focus.

Serotonin deficiency is correlated with depression, low self-esteem, sleep problems, worry, and irritability. A wide range of medications called *antidepressants* are used to treat clinical depression. These meds have varying effects on serotonin, norepinephrine, and dopamine. These same drugs help not only with depression but with mood swings and some obsessive-compulsive disorders. If your dark moods are caused by underlying metabolic disorders, antidepressants can generally work to stabilize your moods. New drugs are continually developed and tested; your doctor can give you the latest information.

Your psychiatrist can determine whether your depression may benefit from antidepressants, as well as the type of medication and dosage you need. (Psychologists are not licensed to prescribe medications, so if you're seeing such a doctor, she may team up with a psychiatrist to make sure that you get the prescription you need.) Table 10-2 lists some common antidepressants.

Table 10-2		Common Antidepressants		
Pharmacological Name	*Brand Names*	*How It Works*	*Pros*	*Cons*
SSRI (Selective Serotonin Reuptake Inhibitors)	Zoloft, Prozac, Luvox, Paxil	Stabilizes serotonin levels.	They reportedly have fewer side effects, and no withdrawal symptoms. Thus, they are generally the first choice of most physicians.	Some media reports have implicated Prozac with mood disturbances and violent behavior, but evidence remains inconclusive. Drug can be transferred in breast milk.

Pharmacological Name	Brand Names	How It Works	Pros	Cons
TCA (Tricyclic Antidepressants)	Adapin, Endep, Norpramin, Pamelor, Sinequan	Thought to increase the brain's levels of norepi-nephrine, a neuro-transmitter.	May be more effective for some patients.	Can cause heat sensitivity. Can cause the body to have difficulty adapting to temperature changes. Must be discontin-ued slowly, or withdrawal symptoms may occur.
MAOI (Monoamine Oxidase Inhibitors)	Nardil, Parnate	Increases levels of epinephrine, norepineph-rine, and serotonin in the brain.	May be effective in cases where patient fails to respond to other medications.	Must adhere to a strict dietary regime: Failure to do so can be fatal. Many other medica-tions react badly with MAOIs.

Bear in mind that relief may not come immediately. You may get lucky and, right off the bat, find what works for you. If not, you may need to go through a trial-and-error period before settling on the right medication and dosage. This process may take a month or longer.

It's fun to mix and match clothes, but you definitely don't want to recklessly combine drugs. Drugs and herbs can have serious interactions with other medications. Tell your doctor about any-thing you're taking, including vitamins, herbs, and supplements. Remember: Combination lunches may be an option in Chinese restaurants, but don't combine prescriptions without asking your doctor!

Be aware that, while these drugs are touted as safe, they have mul-tiple side effects, and the long-term effects on the brain and body have not yet been fully evaluated. It's too soon to say with certainty that the most popular *psychotropic drugs* (drugs that act on your mind) on the market today are completely safe over the long haul.

So you think you're in a rat race . . .

In a study published by the American Psychological Association, Rod K. Dishman, MD, of the University of Georgia used rats to compare exercise to the antidepressant drug imipramine. First, he induced a depression-like condition in these rats by using the drug clomipramine. Then he gave one group of rats 24-hour access to a running-wheel for 12 weeks, but no antidepressants. Another group ran on a treadmill for an hour a day, six days a week for 12 weeks. A third group received imipramine for the last six days of the experiment, and a fourth group received no treatment or exercise.

Dr. Dishman determined whether the rats experienced an improvement in depression by detecting an increase in brain concentration of norepinephrine and serotonin metabolism, and an increase in sexual activity. The rats given imipramine and both exercise groups showed the telltale changes in the balance of neurotransmitters. But only the wheel-running rats showed both an improvement in their mood and an increase in sexual activity.

The moral? Exercise is good; exercise that's not forced is even better. (How's your sex life, by the way?)

Taking a swing at your mood

The same drugs that treat clinical depression can also help with mood swings, one of the key symptoms of hypoglycemia. When your blood sugar is erratic — rising fast in response to eating, then dropping too low shortly after — your moods are likely to swing wildly too. Antidepressants generally work to stabilize your mood. When you get your mood under control, you'll be in a better position to control your diet.

Discussing dietary plans

No matter what you do, if hypoglycemia is the root cause of your depression or cravings, you have to change your diet — no way around that! For instance, a woman in her 40s sought help from various therapists because she'd suffered from depression all her life. The therapists were able to help clear up many long-standing problems, but the depression didn't budge. Finally, they discovered that she had low blood sugar. When she changed her eating habits, her dark moods promptly went away.

Some of the older antidepressants can increase sugar cravings, so tell your doctor that you need to avoid sweets. The newer antidepressant drugs don't have this side effect.

Part V
Spinning a Network of Support for Yourself

The 5th Wave   By Rich Tennant

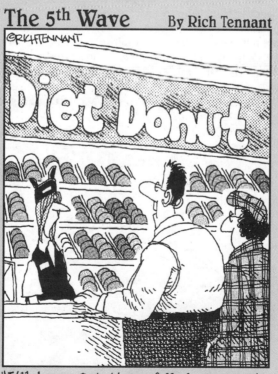

"I'll have 2 lettuce filled, 3 carrot glazed, 5 celery frosted,..."

In this part . . .

Whoever said no man is an island to himself, certainly got it right. Everyone needs the support of other people from time to time; none of us can make it completely alone. In this part, we show you how to set up a support network so that you don't fall on your feet while you're dealing with the side effects and aftereffects of hypoglycemia. After all, everyone is bound to suffer at times from low moods and self-doubts. When you're feeling down, you can open the book to this section and discover how to get through those trying times.

Chapter 11

Jockeying for Support

• •

In This Chapter

▶ Taking a self-inventory for your needs

▶ Getting friends and family to support you

▶ Establishing support groups and buddies

• •

Friends and family help you live longer. Or maybe they just make you feel like you live longer; either way, it works. The fact is, humans are naturally social creatures — homo sapiens would never have survived without banding together in groups. In many, many ways, everyone is dependent on everyone else. (Yes, even you, Mr. Macho Man.)

Now this little exercise isn't the least bit scientific (so don't quote us or shoot us), but think about what low blood sugar could mean metaphorically: Sugar and sweets often symbolize love. So perhaps you can link low blood sugar to lack of love (if you're in love, and your partner has hypoglycemia, check out Chapter 14), or at least to the perception that you're not getting the tender loving care that you need. Perhaps you're surrounded by loving people, but you've walled yourself off from their love. Maybe you need to mend some rifts in your relationships, or maybe you need to establish new relationships. Aside from the physiological basis for addictions, a craving for sugar can mean a craving for love. (By the way, we're not suggesting that a high blood sugar level means that you're getting too much love — it means that you have sugar in your blood, but your cells aren't getting their share. So with both conditions, you're being effectively starved of fuel.)

 Whatever your situation, you need review your health and relationship history if you want to get your blood sugar under control. A growing body of social and scientific evidence points to the vital importance of social contact in the maintenance of your health.

You can start by first reviewing your health history. (Chapter 3 shows you how to observe your symptoms.) Then jot down the names of all your important relationships. This list should include family members, lovers, friends, teachers, and social contacts that are significant to you. No need to write long essays — unless you enjoy that — a few well-chosen words will do. Write down how you feel about these people and your interactions with them. It may also be fun, if you're feeling ambitious, to see if there's any connection between the foods you eat and the people you hang out with. Maybe your mother loves to eat, and she always entices you to eat forbidden foods. Or maybe your ex-boyfriend loved to tempt you with chocolates.

Getting Yourself Out There

What if you live alone? What if you work 12-hour days and are too pooped to go out? Perhaps everyone dearest to you lives in another state or even another country. Go ahead, reach out to them and call them regularly. Make yourself — and your phone company — happy.

If you don't have a family — even a far-flung one — and you don't have a social network, take immediate action to start getting connected to people. Start by getting involved with

- Community organizations (such as the YMCA)
- Social groups sponsored by your particular house of worship
- Classes that interest you (as opposed to those that don't interest you)
- Workshops and seminars
- Volunteer activities
- Professional or trade associations
- Support groups for hypoglycemics (more on this later in this chapter)
- Health or fitness groups

You can find information about these types of groups in your local newspaper or on the Internet.

Get a pet if you can, especially if you live alone and feel isolated. You can get a cat, dog, rabbit, lizard, parakeet, finch, goldfish, or whatever . . . anything that you can love and enjoy taking care of. Studies show that owning and caring for a pet can not only relieve isolation but it can also reduce family arguments and lead to lower levels of anxiety and depression and fewer illnesses.

You may be wondering how any of this relates to low blood sugar. It does! Because to properly treat yourself, you need to look at every aspect of your life. Hypoglycemia is often called a *lifestyle illness*. Its treatment depends more on your diet and lifestyle than on medication or any medical, surgical, or high-tech interventions.

Now go show your family how much you love them — or go grow more branches on your social network.

Getting to Know Me

First things first. Get your food program in order (see Chapter 6). Then write down exactly how you'd like to feel and figure out ways to rearrange your life to best support your journey back to health. (Chapters 16 and 17 offer ideas to get you started.) For this purpose, sit down and have a get-acquainted-with-yourself session. You can have this session alone or with someone you trust.

If you decide to have a get-acquainted-with-yourself session with someone at your side, make sure that you choose someone who's trustworthy and supportive of you. You don't need negativity, criticism, or put-downs. ("Oh hell, honey, you don't have blood sugar problems, you just need a brain transplant.")

1. **Get a notebook and write down everything you're going to do to get healthy.**

   ✔ Physical goals

   - How would you like to look and feel right now?

   - How is your health?

   ✔ Diet

   - Are you keeping a food journal? (See Chapter 6.)

   - Are you keeping track of what foods you should eat and what foods you should avoid? (See Chapter 7 for a list.)

   ✔ Vitamins, supplements, and herbs

   - What vitamins and supplements are you taking?

   - In what quantity are you taking them?

   ✔ Medication

   - What medications are you taking?

   - In what quantity are you taking them?

- Are you setting up and keeping appointments with healthcare practitioners and therapists?

✔ Exercise plan

- What are your current measurements (chest, waist, hips, and so on)?
- What is your current weight?

✔ Meditation, relaxation, and deep breathing

- How often are you meditating?
- How long do your sessions last?

2. **Write exactly how the symptoms caused by your low blood sugar have affected you in each of the following areas:**

- Health (see Chapter 3)
- Family
- Relationships
- Work/Career (see Chapter 12)
- Short- and long-term goals
- Leisure activities

3. **Write how you can avoid the problems caused by your symptoms.**

✔ Health and energy level

- Exercises (see Chapter 8)
- Meditation/breathing (see Chapter 10)
- Herbs, vitamins, and supplements (see Chapter 7)

✔ Job (see Chapter 12)

- How can you manage your symptoms at work?

✔ Managing your moods (Chapter 10)

- Should you consider antidepressants?
- How can you deal with anger?

4. **Write what you think life will be like when you're free of major symptoms.**

✔ Family

- How much time are you spending with your family?
- How can you and your family have more fun together?

✔ Relationship goals

- What would you like your significant relationship to be like?
- What can you do to achieve your ideal relationship?

✔ Support system choice

- What can you do to develop new friendships?
- How can you find groups with similar health goals?

✔ Spiritual needs

- What are you doing to meet your needs? Religious/spiritual practices? Groups? Literature?
- How can you deepen your relationship with others who have a similar spiritual bent?

✔ Career goals

- How do you feel about your job? Are you satisfied?
- Where would you like to be? How will you achieve your goal?

✔ Educational goals

- Are you in school? Do you want to enroll in school?
- What would you like to accomplish?

✔ Others goals or concerns

- Do you want to start a new hobby?
- Do you want to improve another area of life that isn't listed here?

Choose three goals that you want to reach within the next year. Pick something that's easily attainable so that you can get a sense of accomplishment. Every month, review what you've written so that you can see how your objectives or perspectives may have changed. Note if you're feeling more satisfied with life in general as your health improves.

Don't pull the trigger

When it comes to hypoglycemia, what most often derails a treatment program? Food! Food is the biggie, all right. So sit down and brainstorm on all the triggers that can fire your craving for forbidden foods. Write down every single trigger — things, people, or situations that can set off bad eating — that you can think of.

Triggers can be social situations, going to restaurants, losing your pet goldfish, winning the lottery, and so on. Under each trigger, write down what you can do to avoid getting derailed. Go on, wow everyone's socks off with your creative solutions. (For tips and ideas, see Chapters 16 and 17.)

Involving the Whole Fam Damily

If your life has been sweet and sour — you have a sour disposition from eating too many sweets — now is a good time to add a different flavor. How do reconciliation and communication taste to you? How do they taste to your partner, children, parents, or best friend?

Chapter 14 is written just for your significant other. The information in there can help the love of your life make the leap to true partner. Chapter 13 talks more about the following topics in depth.

Can we talk?

You want to involve the whole family, you've got to talk. Set aside a time to talk. Make the occasion relaxing by pouring some herbal tea and playing soft music. Tell your loved ones that you'd like to have a heart-to-heart talk about an important matter.

✔ Embrace your sweetheart or family members and make up for whatever nasty behavior your hypoglycemia caused. Maybe you've let your significant other feel very much insignificant.

- Explain that a lot of the bad stuff — outbursts, fights, and misunderstandings — was due to the effects of low blood sugar.

- Accept full responsibility for your actions.

✔ Get your loved ones to understand the sincerity of your intentions to redirect your lifestyle.

✔ Help your loved ones understand your hypoglycemia.

- Teach them about hypoglycemia and faulty glucose metabolism.

- Read them passages from this book.

- Create a list that describes who you are and what you're going through as you deal with your hypoglycemia (see "Getting to Know Me," earlier in this chapter). Sometimes people understand things better when they're written down.

When can we eat?

Family functions often center around food. Think of the major holidays and special events from your life: cake on your birthday and turkey on Thanksgiving, not to mention all those summer barbecues and late nights ordering pizza. Then you have the daily grind. Someone has to cook dinner. Mac and cheese, anyone?

After talking with your family about what you're experiencing, tell them what you need in terms of food. For more information about food and diet, check out Chapter 6.

- ✔ Tell them that you need to eat certain foods, avoid some foods, and eat frequently.

- ✔ Explain that you need their help in sticking to your food plan. This may involve them reminding you to eat at appropriate times or helping with the preparation of the proper foods.

- ✔ Set boundaries when it comes to what you don't want from them. For instance, you don't need anyone to lay a guilt trip on you.

- ✔ Write down a list of items for your diet and go grocery shopping with your spouse or other willing family members.

- ✔ If you're not the house chef, sit down with the cook and explain all your dietary requirements. Make a copy of your requirements so that they can be referred to easily. You can also offer to take turns cooking, if you aren't already doing so. Or you may want to cook together sometimes.

When your loved one won't help

What if your spouse won't cooperate with your food needs? Well, for starters, you may want to consider couples counseling! Meanwhile, get some help from good friends and a support group. Consult an online hypoglycemia support group (see Chapter 17) for suggestions on what you can do when family members won't help. You may also want to use your support group for developing relationships.

Do you have kiddies? Use this time to wean them off junk foods. They'll probably moan about not being able to eat the foods that all their friends are eating. However, don't force them to give up everything they like. As long as the bulk of their meals are wholesome, and they don't have special health problems requiring a particular diet, you shouldn't be overly strict. Simply stick with your own diet. When you become fit, strong, and energetic — and oh so much more balanced emotionally — they may become so impressed that they'll want to follow the example you set.

WARNING!

Avoiding cults

While you're in a physically and psychologically vulnerable state as a result of your hypoglycemia, having some guidelines can help clarify matters. If you managed to estrange everyone around you and are desperate to be admitted to a group — any group — the possible danger rings even more true. And if it's anything like the first time you felt accepted and cared for, you're wide open for manipulation.

So what's a cult? Having a doctrine doesn't make a group of people a cult. Even claiming that drinking your own urine will heal you of hypoglycemia doesn't make a group of people a cult. (That just makes 'em wacky.) While we have no hard and fast rules for what officially constitutes a cult, watch out for certain signs. The following list provides some signs you should be on the lookout for. The list isn't comprehensive, and not every cult displays all of these characteristics, but if you notice even a few of these signs, consider them a red flag.

- The group has a pyramid-type, authoritarian leadership structure.

- They claim to be the only way to truth, happiness, and healing from hypoglycemia or whatever else ails you.

- They use mind-control techniques on their members that may include subtle brainwashing to make members feel that they're the special "chosen" ones or that the outside world is evil and dangerous.

- They use intimidation, such as belittling or actual threats of violence, to keep members in line.

- They discourage or attempt to cut off your relationships with family and friends.

- They believe that they are right and everyone else is wrong.

- They pressure you to give all that you can to the group — all your money and possessions, for instance.

If you find yourself involved in a group like this, run, don't walk! Cut off all contact with them. It's easier to do so at the first warning sign than after you've been involved for a long time. Don't succumb to pressure to return. Go to a therapist who is knowledgeable about cults. Enlist the support of your family.

TIP

You can change cooking from a chore to a big, fun family affair. One family, for instance, planned everything so that they could cook enough food to last an entire month. (Hey, what are freezers for?) They chose a day when they could all go grocery shopping together. When they finished shopping, they lugged a humongous amount of food to the car. They went wild the following day, cooking batch after batch of wonderful food. Everyone chipped in, including the kids.

If you shudder at the thought of preparing a month's worth of meals, you can fix food for a few days or a week or two. When hunger comes knocking at the door (actually, it shouldn't if you eat regularly like you're supposed to), you won't be tempted to gnaw at the forbidden when you have a delectable and healthy meal readily available.

Joining the In-Crowd

Because humans are social creatures, support groups give you the motivation to stick with a program that's not always easy. Over the long term, members of a group are often much better at accomplishing their goals. Go to local community centers or call hospitals to find groups specific to hypoglycemia. Chapter 17 provides a list of Web sites and other places to contact for such groups.

TIP

Admittedly, groups for hypoglycemia aren't as plentiful as those for other ailments. If you can't find a hypoglycemia-specific group, sign up for groups that have informational or support meetings about health and healing.

Or why not organize your own support group for hypoglycemia? If you get involved with starting a support group, you may find it easier to feel motivated. Okay, get the ball rolling! Don't get bogged down in details. You don't have to wait until you find an ideal meeting place for the group.

1. **Call up everyone you know who might be interested in joining a support group for hypoglycemia.**

   Ask friends, neighbors, and colleagues if they are interested in joining your group. You can also ask them if they know anyone else who may have low blood sugar.

2. **Put up flyers and ads promoting your group.**

3. **Start your own Web site or newsletter.**

4. **Decide on a meeting place.**

   You can find a meeting place at the homes of members or at libraries and bookstores. You can usually meet at libraries and bookstores for free, and they may be more accessible for drop-ins. You may even be able to get a group discount by purchasing books on hypoglycemia or other related subjects at bookstores where you frequently meet.

5. **Consider charging a membership fee.**

   Discuss what you think is a fair amount to charge participants. You'll want to be able to cover expenses plus have some money left over for other purposes, such as inviting speakers or financing creative events. Charging a membership fee for the group will make people value it more. Freebies just can't get respect. (This is the same idea used to set the prices for doctor's and lawyer's fees and expensive cosmetics that probably don't cost more than a dollar to produce.)

Netting some help

Finding online support groups — those you can contact through the Internet — for hypoglycemics may be easier than finding groups that meet in person. Key phrases to enter into a search

REMEMBER

Eat before you type

It can be all too easy to spend hours surfing the Internet. Before you go online, make sure that you eat something. You may want to set a timer or alarm clock to remind you to eat your next snack or meal. Keeping your blood sugar regulated is important. You don't want to get irritated and send nasty messages that you later regret. Some otherwise sweet people can undergo a sudden transformation and lash out at nothing in particular when their blood sugar is low. After they eat and restore themselves to sanity, they then spend an inordinate amount of time apologizing to the hapless recipients of their e-mail. If this pattern of behavior sounds familiar, post a reminder note by your computer: Eat before you write. Don't send messages when annoyed.

Just because you don't see anyone's face (unless you have a Web camera), and you can hide behind your computer screen, you don't have a license to be rude. Extend the same courtesy you show when interacting face to face. Don't spread rumors, send unsolicited ads, or insult people. Everyone is entitled to their opinion. And when you're involved with support groups, all of your personal information should be kept confidential.

engine are **hypoglycemia, support groups,** or **low blood sugar.** You can find numerous online support groups where you can discuss any issues you're working through. (Flip to Chapter 17 for resources.)

For those of you who spend a great part of your time in front of the computer already, try to participate in real flesh-and-blood groups in addition to, or in lieu of, online support. You can't substitute for face-to-face experience. But chat groups, message boards, and e-mails are convenient ways to contact people. You may also be able to develop a good rapport with people online.

And now a word to the wise. You should be careful when you post messages online. We're not talking Big Brother here, but unlike the spoken word, your written words do get stored, and the chance exists that someone, somewhere can use it against you. It's not likely, but a little caution never hurt anyone. Remember, too, that people you meet online can pretend to be anyone they want to be. People can, and do, try on different identities and different genders. Luckily, this practice is much more common in groups devoted to the dating game; most of the people involved in hypoglycemic groups are sincerely engaged in getting their blood sugar levels under control and helping others do the same.

Doing the 12-step

Twelve-step groups help members overcome various addictions by following a series of (surprise!) 12 steps. If you can't find a good hypoglycemic group, and you don't want to start one of your own, twelve-stepping may be the solution for you. (If you're looking for a dance group, try classes.)

Here are some advantages to joining a twelve-step program:

- ✔ They offer support to those who are desperate, whether they take the form of addiction, unhealthy relationship dependencies, or other emotional issues. (Bring plenty of tissues if you tend to get teary-eyed.)

- ✔ Meetings can be found in virtually any community. There seem to be more 12-step groups than other types of support groups. If you'd rather talk face to face, it's better to physically attend a group.

- ✔ You don't have to pay dues or fees. You may make voluntary contributions.

You may feel isolated when trying to deal with your low blood sugar problem. You may feel as though no one else has to face the same challenges. But when you sit in these meetings, you'll most likely come away with the realization that everyone has her own cross to bear. You may also come to realize that when the you-know-what hits the fan, some people will help you clean it up. You're not alone. You can go to weekly meetings, and you can collect telephone numbers and personal contacts if you wish. You can also get a one-on-one sponsor to help you overcome hurdles.

Overeaters Anonymous

If you can't find a group specific to hypoglycemia, Overeaters Anonymous (OA) may be of value. A general misconception is that you have to be overweight to join OA. Not so. Meetings are also available for those suffering with bulimia or anorexia, two eating disorders.

OA focuses on issues with food; it does not necessarily focus on weight loss or advocate any one type of diet. It addresses physical, emotional, and spiritual well-being. OA can be a good choice for hypoglycemics who may have some emotional issues with food. If, no matter what you do, you can't seem to curb your cravings, OA may be a good forum for you. You can share with others the difficulty of trying to adhere to a healthy diet.

Alcoholics Anonymous

Alcoholics Anonymous (AA) is for those who wish to recover from, or are in the process of recovering from, alcoholism. Alcoholism is not unusual in hypoglycemics, because faulty glucose metabolism may be at the root of the addiction in the first place. (See Chapter 2 for more on alcoholism and low blood sugar.) If you have parents who are alcoholics, you're likely to have either drinking problems or hypoglycemia. Or maybe both.

If your drinking is getting out of hand, you should definitely consider following the basic hypoglycemic diet and either enroll yourself in a treatment program for alcoholics or join AA. Sticking to your diet may also help you control your alcohol problems.

Emotions Anonymous

Emotions Anonymous (EA) is for people who have difficulty dealing with their emotions. This group can help you deal with the emotions and mood swings that may be caused, in part, by your erratic blood sugar.

Don't look for medical or psychiatric service from EA groups, and don't expect personal or family counseling. Just like all other twelve-step groups, it's not a professionally run organization, but the famous 12 steps give the group structure and unity.

EA addresses a wide variety of emotional issues, including depression, anger, broken or strained relationships, grief, anxiety, low self-esteem, panic, abnormal fears, resentment, jealousy, guilt, despair, boredom, loneliness, withdrawal, obsessive and negative thinking, worry, and compulsive behavior. (Chapter 3 talks about the symptoms of hypoglycemia.)

Buddying Up

With the buddy system, you pair up with a friend and help each other attain a goal you both want. For instance, you may both want to change your diet. The buddy system works by making you accountable for what you've agreed to do for your own benefit. Cheating or sliding can be all too easy if you're the only one taking account of your actions. When you have a friend that you have to answer to, it somehow becomes much more important to meet your self-imposed goal, which may be to quit eating sugar or start exercising.

When you can't stick to your exercise program, or you're tempted to go off your diet, or you're just having a bad day, phone your buddy. Are you craving sugar because you're lonely, angry, or depressed? Telephone your buddy. Listening to your buddy's problems will help you, as well. In fact, you may begin to form a bond. When your buddy has a success, you'll feel as though you have had a success, as well. Your buddy's success may motivate you to reach your own health goals. When you have someone pulling for you, you don't want to let that person down. And when you're responsible for someone else, you're less likely to cheat.

Who should you pair up with? You can pair up with anyone who has a similar goal or concern, and who you can trust to keep up the alliance. Find someone else who is concerned with low blood sugar. If you can't find someone who has hypoglycemia and would like to work on a recovery program, remember that plenty of people want to lose weight. So pair up with someone who's trying to shed some pounds or cut sugar from his or her diet. Because your goals will be similar, you'll probably work well together. You'll both need to exercise, and many foods that are off-limits for you are also banned from weight-reduction diets. Differences are sure to occur, so you don't need to follow the same diet. Just explain to each other what you intend to do, and make sure that your partner keeps his or her word. You need to be caring and compassionate, but strict. Don't let your partner slip up, and vice versa. Be willing to scold each other in a caring, supportive way.

At the initial meeting between you and your buddy, you need to

✔ Establish a meeting frequency.

- Depending on your schedule, agree to meet weekly or biweekly. You'll lose momentum if you go longer between meetings.

- Determine what you'd like to do during your meetings. Set time aside to meditate together or read quotes from inspirational books.

- Agree on a time when you can call to check up on your progress. Ideally, you should call every day; send an e-mail instead if it will work better for you. It doesn't have to be a long-winded conversation — two to five minutes will suffice for a daily check-in. When you're experiencing difficulties that can throw you off track, you can schedule a longer conversation to discuss it with your buddy.

✔ Establish your goals.

✔ Determine how you'll meet your goals.

✔ Share literature so that you can better understand what the other person needs.

✔ Show your buddy everything you write down in terms of your wants and needs.

✔ Explain your diet and the concept. (See Chapter 6 for diet information.)

✔ When you meet your goals, take turns rewarding each other. You can give each other a massaging, go to a movie or for a hike, or do anything that you find pleasurable. (Don't use food as a reward!) This is one sweet alliance that won't cause your blood sugar to come crashing down.

The downside of the buddy system is the possibility that one or both of you may slip up on your commitments to yourselves and to each other. You can falter despite the best of intentions. Maybe your hypoglycemic symptoms are too much for you to handle; or you have other things going on that are more demanding of your time; or you find that you've paired up with the wrong person. If you slip up, don't despair. Discuss it with your buddy to see if you both would like to give it another shot, change what you're doing, or just drop it. If you decide that the partnership isn't working out, you may want to find someone else.

Chapter 12

Making Sure They Get a Good Eight Hours from You

● ●

In This Chapter

▶ Living with hypoglycemia at work

▶ Informing others of your hypoglycemia

▶ Dealing with long workdays

▶ Handling stressors at work

● ●

*H*aving a metabolic disorder such as hypoglycemia doesn't have to unduly complicate your life. With just a few adjustments and modifications, it can fit into your working life, as well. Taking control over hypoglycemia is all about planning and management.

Make your health a priority. You may think that putting your work first is virtuous and will help you get ahead, but in the long run, you'll only be sabotaging yourself with health problems.

To better manage your health, you may need to let co-workers know about your health challenges. (This doesn't mean coming across as a hypochondriac or someone who's using health issues as an excuse to get special treatment.) This chapter shows you how to inform others of your health concerns in a professional, respectful manner that won't undermine your credibility.

The issue of work stress are also addressed. No matter what type of work you do, you are bound to be confronted with stressors, making it that much more difficult to deal with your hypoglycemic symptoms.

No Rings Around Either: Blue and White Collar Workers

Because there are so many different jobs out there, we can't cover every angle of dealing with hypoglycemia at work. (For work-related legal matters, see "Flying with the legal eagles," later in this chapter.) Whatever your field, whatever your collar color, all jobs offer different challenges, so we can only offer generalities. Only you know the special circumstances and the particulars of your job. It shouldn't be that difficult to accommodate your needs, no matter where you work.

Hard hat area

If you engage in physical labor, you have to be especially careful about your blood sugar level. Symptoms such as tremors of the hand, dizziness, or weakness can jeopardize your safety. It's imperative that you eat something every two hours to maintain a constant blood sugar level.

You need to get enough calories, too. Depending on how vigorous your work is, you may want to eat a lot more carbs. Instead of consuming roughly 40 percent of your calories in carbohydrates, as is normally recommended for hypoglycemics, you can consume up to 60 percent. (Chapter 6 tells you more about percentages and portions.) Start with a small increase in the amount of carbs you eat, and then gradually increase the amount to see how it makes you feel. If the increase triggers more hypoglycemic symptoms and carbohydrate cravings, cut back. Make sure that you're eating only high quality carbs, such as non-starchy veggies and whole grains. Limit bread to one slice a day, and eat more grains such as millet and quinoa. (See Chapter 6 for information about healthy foods.) Be sure to carry snacks with you wherever you go. Never, ever go anywhere without food.

Tie required

If you work regular hours in an office, you should be able to eat every two to two-and-a-half hours during breaks and lunch. If your break times aren't regular, and you often forget to take them because you're concentrating on your work, it may be a good idea to

✔ Set a wristwatch with multiple alarms.

✔ Have a family member or an answering service call you at pre-arranged times.

✔ Make signs for your desk to remind yourself.

To Whom It May Concern: Addressing Your Boss and Co-Workers

Where are you in terms of work? Are you barely holding your own? Is your work record so spotty, that you may be fired? Do you have excessive absenteeism due to your health condition? Or, are you in pretty good shape, just needing a little bit of help from your colleagues to function better?

Depending on your job and your relationship with your superiors, you may be hesitant to approach them with what appears to be a personal problem. You may be especially concerned if your company's corporate culture is cutthroat, and any shortcomings on your part, real or imagined, can be used as ammunition against you. On the other hand, if your health is impacting your work performance, it's not just your problem. You need to work out a solution.

Discuss the matter if you

✔ Work somewhere with a policy against eating at your desk, and you can't get away to a breakroom for a snack

✔ Need extra breaks

✔ Frequently travel for your job

✔ Are expected to put in long hours

✔ Often call in sick

✔ Have been unable to concentrate, and your performance has suffered

You may want to discuss matters with Human Resources (HR) before approaching your boss, as HR usually has to clear any special arrangements. Of course, if you have a wonderful rapport with your boss, you may want to go to her first; it helps to have someone on your side.

Bad work habits don't just include surfing the Internet

Here are some things that will stress you out, unbalance you physically, mentally, and emotionally, and ultimately lead to problems with blood sugar regulation:

- Skipping breakfast

- Skipping lunch

- Shoveling food into your mouth

- Not taking enough breaks

- Continuing to work when exhausted

- Staying up late to finish the day's work

- Being a perfectionist

- Exposing yourself to toxic household products (See the resources in Chapter 17 to find out where you can purchase safe products.)

- Making negative comments to yourself, like "No one appreciates the work I do."

- Failing to communicate with colleagues

- Not trusting others to do their share of the work

- Needing to validate your self-worth through work

- Not asking for help when you need it

- Refusing to acknowledge that hypoglycemia is a problem that needs to be treated

To discover how to better manage yourself, turn to Chapters 9 and 16.

Remember that you have certain rights, and if your health is a matter that needs to be discussed, by all means, do so. You may have more credibility if you get a diagnosis from a medical doctor or other healthcare practitioner before coming out as a hypoglycemic.

If your condition is not very severe, and it hasn't impacted your work, then perhaps you don't need to mention it to your supervisor. Consider all your options and your particular situation. You know where you are in the corporate hierarchy (assuming that you work for a corporation) and what your corporate culture is like. If it's a nice, cozy family-like atmosphere, you may have little to worry about; although there are fewer work places like that today.

Find at least one ally at work who is caring, trustworthy, and dependable. If you can't trust yourself to eat regularly, and you can't make any other arrangements, perhaps you can ask this person to remind you to do so until your condition improves. As an adult, it may seem weird to ask someone to remind you to eat. You're not in kindergarten, after all! But the point is that when your brain isn't getting its fuel, your thinking function starts to shut down. When your thinking shuts down, you probably aren't going to remember when you have to eat. Explain the physical condition that you have; emphasize that it won't be a permanent arrangement. When your condition stabilizes, you'll be in good enough shape that you won't need these constant reminders.

Normally, you should be able to snack at regularly scheduled breaks and lunch. If you find that you need to eat more often, and your employer has a "no eating at the desk" policy, gently ask your supervisor for special permission because of your physical condition.

Flying with the legal eagles

Before talking to your supervisor, it may be helpful to become familiar with your rights as an employee, especially as they pertain to your health. The Americans with Disabilities Act (ADA) protects your rights as an employee if you are "a qualified individual with disabilities." Who falls under this category? Anyone with a physical or mental impairment that substantially limits one or more major life activities, such as seeing, hearing, speaking, walking, breathing, performing manual tasks, learning, caring for oneself, and working. These disabilities include such conditions as epilepsy, paralysis, HIV infection, and diabetes. Sprains, broken limbs, or the flu won't cut it.

In other words, even if you tell your employer that you have hypoglycemia, they can't fire you on the basis of that alone. You have the right to ask your employer for any reasonable accommodations you need to perform the duties assigned to you. Of course, what's reasonable is open to interpretation, but if both parties are acting in good faith, you should be able to work out an arrangement that's satisfactory for everyone concerned.

To protect yourself, you should follow these steps:

1. **Get a letter or memo, preferably from a medical doctor, explaining your illness.**

   If you can't get the note from a doctor, get it from another health practitioner. Ask for a written diagnosis and medical recommendations. At the very least, try to obtain a written description of your condition for your employer's benefit. Go to someone who's familiar with your symptoms and can confirm the dates you suffered and the specific symptoms.

2. **Ask to speak to your supervisor about your condition privately.**

   If the situation warrants it, you may want to wait until the end of the work day to discuss the matter. Be forthright about your physical condition, as your supervisor needs to be aware of your symptoms.

3. **Keep a written record of any communication between yourself and management, including the date(s) of your meeting with your supervisor and what you talked about.**

You may need to prove that you did your best to work things out, so it's important to create a paper trail. Don't announce that you're keeping a file, however. If the meeting with your supervisor does not go well, don't discuss it with anyone else in the office, as people may think that you're complaining about management. You don't want to appear as if you're being antagonistic.

This list assumes that nothing drastic has happened so far. If things have already gotten out of hand, and you have received disciplinary action, you can ask to see what's in your file. It's important to find out what is in your file so that you can figure out what to do. If the information is accurate, try to correct any work problems that have been pointed out. If the information is inaccurate, find a way to correct it. Check with your union steward (if you have one) to see how you can do this.

Framing your condition in a positive way

When speaking to your supervisor or management about your condition, follow these simple guidelines:

✓ **Be honest.** Simply state that hypoglycemia is a condition that's related to diabetes, and that you've been advised that it may progress into diabetes if you don't treat it properly. Therefore, you're acting in a responsible manner by taking whatever measures are necessary to prevent your condition from becoming more of a problem.

One caveat: Don't feel compelled to give a blow-by-blow account of every pain and ache you have. Keep the discussion brief and to the point.

✔ **Apologize immediately for any problems or inconveniences that your symptoms may have caused.** Your tone should be one of taking responsibility, not of self-pity or complaint. You don't want to make yourself sound like a hopeless invalid.

✔ **Accept input about where you may have fallen short in your work performance as a result of your physical condition.** If he gives no such input, simply point out things you'll do to make sure that your work improves.

✔ **Don't dwell on the problem.** Whatever your challenges, ruminating on them will only make you feel worse. You're more likely to come up with creative solutions if you take a break from thinking about your problem.

✔ **Focus on the positives, not the negatives.** Because you have become more knowledgeable about your condition and are participating in a healthy lifestyle, you can be even more productive than other employees. To effectively live with hypoglycemia, you have to be self-disciplined, self-aware, and self-responsible — all of these are invaluable characteristics that companies look for in their employees.

✔ **Emphasize that you know what the problem is and you're getting a handle on it.** When you learn to control the problem, your condition will stabilize, and you'll fulfill the essential tasks of your employment position.

If you frame requests in a positive way, you'll be more likely to be heard. At the least, it'll keep any discussions from turning ugly. Keep in mind that your employer hired you to carry out a specific job; you have an obligation and responsibility to fulfill your duties to the best of your ability.

Finding practical solutions

Before you approach your boss, make a list of the topics you want to discuss and the specific requests you're making. Prepare alternatives for whatever requests you're making.

Bring the supervisor into the process of finding solutions. Be open to her suggestions, but don't put the onus on her to come up with ideas. Make it clear that you're on the same side, trying to find ways to help you be as productive as possible at work.

✔ **Offer general information about hypoglycemia's symptoms and how you can prevent them.** An understanding of the condition and the possible need for regular work schedules and meal breaks is usually helpful and appreciated.

✔ **Keep a progress report for yourself.** That way, if necessary, you can point out that you're following through on your commitment to work things out responsibly.

✔ **Talk privately to co-workers that you may have offended with your mood swings or temper outbursts.** Tell them what low blood sugar can do to one's brain. It may take a little time, but after you show that you're getting more stable, they may be ready to trust you.

✔ **Eat a small snack before meetings so that you don't have a sudden blood sugar dip.** Even with such precautions, people with a blood sugar imbalance may feel fine one minute and then, suddenly, without warning, feel faint or weak the next. If you're prone to such attacks, bring something to drink with you, such as milk, soy milk, or fruit juice diluted with water. These drinks should be enough to forestall a hypoglycemic incident. If you still have problems, ask your supervisor if you can leave briefly to get a snack.

Putting Up a Cot in the Cubicle? Managing Long Work Hours

Do you work more than 40 hours a week? Surveys show that a rising number of people in the United States are clocking in a record number of hours at work. It's not uncommon for people to put in 18 to 20 hours a day. In fact, Americans are pulling in longer hours than most other nations, surpassing even workaholic Japan! We're talking about averages here, of course. Your country of residence doesn't preclude you from working inordinately long hours. It all depends on individual circumstances.

If you want to work efficiently, figure out your personal rhythm and try to work in accordance with it. Different occupations have different rhythms, tempos, and paces. If your natural rhythm isn't in accordance with your job's rhythm, you'll likely wear yourself out.

Ask yourself the following questions:

✔ Am I a morning person or a night owl? (Hypoglycemics tend to do better at night, although there are exceptions.)

✔ Do I work better or worse under deadline pressure?

✔ Do I work in spurts, or at an even, constant pace?

Now, ask the following questions in relation to your work:

✔ Am I a team player or a lone wolf?

✔ Which tasks do I enjoy the most?

✔ Which tasks give me the most problems?

Consider tackling the most troublesome portion of your job when you're the most energetic, and reward yourself with the tasks that you truly enjoy. If there's nothing about your work that you like, make plans to get into a different line of work. Even if it means working toward a distant goal, taking concrete action should make your current circumstances easier.

✔ **Take a mini break every 45 to 60 minutes.** (This is in addition to the official 10 to 15 minute breaks you may get.)

 • Do a few neck rolls and eye rolls, and let your eyes rest by looking out into the distance.

 • Make sure that you blink frequently if you work on a computer for most of the day. (The person who blinks first is *not* the loser.)

 • Do a few *isometrics* (exercises in which you contract certain muscles). For instance, tighten your thigh muscles for a few seconds and then release.

 • Stretch out a little every once in a while. Go to the water cooler or the bathroom.

Don't worry, you're not wasting time. All it takes is a few minutes. It'll make a big difference in your performance and the way you feel. Your focus, concentration, and thinking will be much sharper.

You may, at times, feel more lethargic or cloudy headed than usual. Or you may notice an increase in the intensity of some of your other symptoms. To help alleviate your symptoms, try to schedule your main breaks so that you can physically lie down for 15 minutes (or for a half an hour during lunch). Lying down is much more restorative than sitting. If lying down is just not possible, perhaps you can put your head down on your desk and close your eyes. Even resting with your head down on your desk can make a world of difference.

✔ **Eat every 1½ to 2 hours.** (This is especially important for maintaining your blood sugar.) You won't lose any time. We're not talking a banquet here. You can snack while you're working.

✔ **Eat more protein for lunch.** When you start on your hypoglycemic diet, you may begin to notice that you don't have post-lunch drowsiness and mid-afternoon slumps like you used to. If you still have problems, cut back drastically on starches such as pasta and grains.

✔ **Work out at least three times a week.** Don't become a weekend warrior who crams in hours of exercise on days off. This type of behavior is excellent — for heart attacks.

✔ **At the end of the day or on days off, allow yourself to rest without guilt.**

- Get other members of the family to do household chores, such as cleaning or the laundry. Or hire help.

- Eat out instead of cooking at home (if you think it will help). Just make sure that you order something within your diet plan, such as salad, steamed vegetables, and grilled fish or chicken.

✔ **Ask yourself if you really need to work all those hours.** Keep a written record of all your activities during the day. When you review the account, you'll be able to see where the time wasters are, what can be eliminated or reduced, and where you can improve efficiency. The idea is to work smarter, not harder.

Diffusing Work-Related Stress

Work has stresses all its own — stresses different from those in your personal life. Isn't that nice? Here's how you can deal with these special stresses.

✔ **It may sound trite, but live one day at a time.** When something goes wrong at work, remind yourself that this too shall pass. Will anyone care about it a hundred years from now? Will *you* care about it in a year?

✔ **Eliminate the stressors that can be avoided, and learn to handle everyday stress through meditation and exercise.** (See Chapter 9 for info on how to reduce stress.) Remember that managing stress is a big part of attaining and maintaining health.

✔ **Go away for a mini-retreat if you can.** Take an entire weekend off where you won't be interrupted and can have time to relax and do a major life review. Where are you in your career right now? Where do you want to be? Should you quit your current job? Play for a promotion? Go into a different line of work? Go back to school? Write your memoir? Become a mime?

✔ **Have fun.** This may not be on your radar screen when you're overworked, but it's important to schedule some fun time into every day, even if it's for 10 minutes. Have lunch with someone you enjoy. Go window shopping. Read the funnies. Sketch a drawing. Call up a friend and shoot the breeze. At least once a week, try to do something pleasurable that takes a couple of hours or more. For extra enjoyment and relaxation, get a weekly massage if you can afford it. If not, trade massages with family or friends. It's all about inner and outer balance.

Now, if your work is seriously detracting from your quality of life and contributing to your poor health, you should take this opportunity to do a major life review. If you're in poor health, or you're having a constellation of symptoms (maybe even a galaxy of them), something's not right, whether it's physical, mental, emotional, or spiritual. Your body's metabolic imbalance may be a reflection of an imbalance in your life. To become completely well, you're going to have to address your health in a multi-faceted way, physically, mentally, emotionally, and spiritually. Work occupies most of our waking time; how healthy can you become if your job is a source of major dissatisfaction? The stress of doing work you're not suited for can only exacerbate your hypoglycemia.

The 6:00 unwind

It's hard to unwind after working a stressful day. Be careful, because overwork can cause your adrenals to become overactive and hypervigilant, thus triggering panic attacks. To relax, instead of reaching for a stiff drink — which is taboo for hypoglycemics — try doing a gentle yoga routine, deep breathing, or meditation. Take a long, relaxing bath with epsom salts. Listen to some music and read a good book. It has been discovered that watching TV or getting on the computer at night can interefere with sound sleep. And when you're working more than normal, you need to get as deep and restful a sleep as possible. In order to get restorative sleep at night, sleep in a dark room or wear eye shades. Remove all electrical appliances with flashing lights from your bedroom; these appliances have been shown to impede deep sleep.

It's probably wise to postpone making any major decisions until you have your diet under control and your symptoms have abated. It's hard to make sound decisions when your thinking is fuzzy and you're not functioning very well. You can get at least some of your symptoms under control through herbs and supplements. (For a list of herbs and supplements, refer to Chapter 7.) If your main problem is anxiety and depression, and natural remedies aren't helping, try medication. (To read about anxiety and depression, and medicine's role in treating these conditions, turn to Chapter 10.)

Of course, only you can decide what the best course of action is. If you love your job, or you desperately need the income, sit down and figure out exactly how you need to change your work arrangement. If a reasonable effort to change things on your part meets with no results, you and your job may have to part ways. Make sure that you get yourself a parachute before you take that leap, though! Not having a job can be very stressful.

Passing up the go juice

Java. The bean. Joe. Whatever you call it, it seems that everybody is drinking coffee in the morning.

Caffeine is detrimental to hypoglycemics. If you're addicted to coffee (you get a headache when you've gone a while without a mug, even if you only drink a cup a day), taper your use gradually. If you try to stop cold turkey, you'll get a headache. The following list provides some good ways to help you make the transition from coffee to some healthy alternatives:

- **Find good caffeine-free coffee substitutes.** These may include grain coffees or herbal teas.

- **Drink green tea or herbal tea.** You may want to try Japanese barley tea (mugi-cha), which doesn't have caffeine.

- **Make a protein smoothie with protein powder, or create your own favorite drink.**

- **Mix up some hot chocolate with carob powder and nut or rice milk, and add some stevia to sweeten.** *Carob,* a natural chocolate substitute, doesn't contain stimulants. It also helps normalize hypoglycemia.

If you absolutely must drink some coffee

- **Don't drink coffee on an empty stomach.** It can be very hard on your stomach; besides, it really creates havoc on your blood sugar.

✔ **Drink coffee with lots of cream.** The protein and fat in the cream will help stabilize your blood sugar (somewhat) and mitigate the negative effects of the caffeine. (Remember, cream does add calories.)

✔ **Take extra B complex tabs.** Coffee is believed to deplete the vitamin B in your system. If you just can't resist tasting coffee, take a few sips and leave the rest.

Need a quick pick-me-up? Well then, take deep, uncaffeinated breaths. You can go to the bathroom or the lounge and meditate for a few minutes, too. Or, if it's during your official break time or lunch, go outside and run around the building. If you have enough time, you may even decide to go to the gym. But don't skip your lunch to do so.

Creating a cozy cubicle

Cubicles are just as much a part of some working cultures as coffee drinking. Most people spend the majority of their waking time at work, so you should create as healthy and as pleasant an environment as you can.

✔ Do you have a co-worker who always sets out a bowl of candies for everyone? To avoid temptation, don't even get close to it. Make sure that you have healthy snacks on hand for just such an occasion.

✔ Office vending machines are bad news. You'll make it easier for yourself if you make them off limits. If there's a healthy food item you want that can be sold through a vending machine, it won't hurt to ask the vending company to carry it. Call up the company directly, or waylay the guy who stocks the machines.

✔ Do they wheel danishes and donuts into your office every morning? If so, find out if they can also start bringing in healthier treats so that people can have a choice. Because so many people are on weight-reducing diets these days, you may find a lot of supporters.

✔ Noise pollution can add to stress, which in turn can exacerbate hypoglycemic symptoms. If the noise in your work environment bothers you, get a white noise generator. These machines can deflect unwanted sounds and mask discordant noise by producing a smooth sound of rushing air that creates a sense of calm. Some of them even produce a variety of low frequency digital sounds, including the sounds of a lakeshore, rain, surf, a brook, a waterfall, and a country evening.

✔ People whose bodies are very sensitive, like most low blood sugar sufferers, are better off using only environmentally sound cleaning products at home and in the office. Some particularly susceptible people may become acutely ill if they work in offices that suffer from *sick building syndrome* (buildings with a high degree of indoor pollution). This often occurs in insulated buildings with windows that don't open. If you discover anything at work that you're quite allergic to, find out how you can avoid being exposed to it.

✔ If the quality of the air in your workplace is a problem, get an air purifier. Keeping plants on your desk can also help; if nothing else, they can enliven your work space.

✔ Music can have the same calming effect as tranquilizers. Play relaxing music while you work. Just make sure that you don't bother your co-workers.

Chapter 13

Dealing with Friends and Family: Eat and Let Eat

In This Chapter

▶ Talking to your loved ones about hypoglycemia

▶ Communicating your needs

▶ Sticking to your diet in the face of naysayers

*T*he world would be fine and splendid if you could always count on those nearest and dearest to you to be your most enthusiastic cheerleaders. They're the ones who exert the most power over you. Yet the sad truth is that, instead of inspiring you, they're often the very ones who drag you down. They may well be good, decent people who have the most honorable intentions, but they can still thwart your attempt to regain your health.

When it comes to hypoglycemia, most people may not be very sympathetic or helpful. Why is this? Well, first of all, regardless of how wretched it may make you feel, hypoglycemia is generally not life threatening. Secondly, people still tend to believe that it's all in your head or that you're just malingering. Perhaps in their opinion you were doing just fine before, so why this sudden and drastic attempt to change?

Your first task, therefore, is to help your loved ones understand this admittedly perplexing syndrome. After they understand it, they may be much more willing to support your recovery process. Then and only then can you proceed to ask them for help in changing your lifestyle and dealing with the symptoms of hypoglycemia. Don't assume that they'll automatically know what to do; you have to let them know exactly what you need from them. Present your requests clearly and directly, and don't place blame on anyone.

This chapter gives you the tools to communicate your wants effectively — specifically in terms of changing your diet — and shows you how to deal with your family. (Hey, this is a book on hypoglycemia!)

'Splaining to Your Schmoopies

It's hard for people who have normal metabolism to understand the energy fluctuations your low blood sugar causes. These fluctuations are one of the first things you need to help your loved ones understand.

To convey information about your condition, take a cue from the politicians:

- ✔ **Prepare your statements in advance so that you don't become confused and forget the important points.**
- ✔ **Collect and present literature about hypoglycemia.**
- ✔ **Try not to look like you're announcing a stock market crash.** A talk doesn't need to be deadly serious. You can be informal but informative. Or, conversely, you can ham it up — go all out and type out written statements for everyone to read. (You can also photocopy some pages from this book.)
- ✔ **Let your loved ones understand that you're nothing if not serious about the lifestyle changes you're going to make.** (Well, aren't you?) But have a sense of humor about it. Don't make it sound as though you're going to do yourself in if your family doesn't do what you want them to do.

The most important points to convey include the following:

- ✔ What hypoglycemia is
- ✔ How important it is to regulate your blood sugar
- ✔ How the wrong foods can contribute to your condition
- ✔ The health impact of a blood sugar imbalance
- ✔ The food plan you need to follow
- ✔ Exercise and other lifestyle changes you'd like to make

Chapters 2, 6, and 8 provide the info everyone needs about the particular topics listed here.

If this list seems like too much to discuss, simply inform your family that you have hypoglycemia and you're making dietary changes. Then show them the list of foods you can and cannot eat.

Helping Them Help You

Your family may ask you right off the bat what they can do to help. Naaaah! That would never happen. It's up to you to ask for help from the people you love most (and who love you most).

- **Ask yourself first what your family can do to help.** (Either that or ask what you can do for your country.) Certain household chores may become difficult for you to do, for example, when paired with other syndromes like fybromyalgia.

- **State your requests clearly and in a matter-of-fact way.** Here's an example: You're the cook, but you find that brain fog interferes with your duties. Give explicit instructions for someone else to make out a shopping list for you. Make it a joint, cooperative venture.

- **Don't turn requests into a threat or a demand.** At the same time, don't sound apologetic.

- **If stress is a problem — and it usually is — figure out how you can tackle it together.** Brainstorm ways to deal with this and other issues.

- **Use "I" statements.** Statements that begin with "I" instead of "you" sound less like accusations. For example, suppose you're hurt because your spouse refuses to support you. You shouldn't say, "You're a real moron for not understanding how important this is to me. You always were a &%*$ [fill in with any of your favorite four-letter words]." A far better approach is, "I feel hurt when you won't listen to my explanations about how food can seriously affect my body chemistry and my ability to function. I tell myself then that you don't care about my health."

- **Don't interrupt, bring up unrelated elements, or change the subject.** Setting ground rules can go a long way toward smoother communication.

- **If a digression occurs, table it.** Digression can bring up significant issues. For instance, when you're trying to communicate the frustrations you experience with hypoglycemia, and your partner complains that you never come through with your promises, you have the chance to point out that it's related to your particular biochemical disorder, and now that you know what's causing these problems, you're bound and determined to change them — and you need all the support you can get.

Repeat or paraphrase what your loved one just said. This approach is also useful if you suffer from brain fog and tend to space out what someone's saying.

✔ **Don't keep your problem to yourself.** You may think that keeping your hypoglycemia to yourself will ensure harmony, but in the long run, it can backfire. Rather than let health problems create difficulties in your relationships, use them as a communication bridge for building a stronger foundation.

✔ **Express appreciation for any support your family gives you.** It's also a good idea to give thanks for specific acts of consideration. For instance, you may want to say, "Timothy, I really am thankful that you agreed to do all the grocery shopping for all of us. It helps me avoid foods I'm not supposed to have."

✔ **Express the love you feel.** Don't bottle it up; spread it around. Show love to your family and friends every day. Spend time having fun with them. Doing so will work wonders with keeping your body chemistry balanced.

Dealing with the Doubting Thomases

You have to get used to it — people giving you grief about your syndrome, that is. A lot of people don't believe that nutrition can have such a profound effect on someone with a sensitive body chemistry. They may think that you're off the wall, and they may accuse you of malingering.

We'd like to tell you to tough it out, pump up your emotional muscles, and deflect verbal punches, but that's much easier said than done, especially when you're feeling unbalanced. Daily exchanges with a doubting Thomas or hostile person can set you back and perhaps drive you to emotional eating, which can then trigger more of your symptoms. Not good.

If your family gives you grief when you speak to them about changing your diet, they may be feeling threatened by the prospect of change. You're tampering with the very foundation of family life — your daily food! If their eating habits are less than healthy, you may be triggering guilt and anxiety. The remedy is to offer a lot of affection and reassure them as much as you can. You can point out that as your blood sugar becomes better regulated and your health improves, you'll be calmer, happier, and more loving.

The best way to deal with doubting Thomases? Don't listen to them. Stop them in their tracks. Refuse to discuss hypoglycemia or related topics with them. You can't convert someone with a heated exchange. Switch the subject. And if they persist, tell them that you don't care to talk about it. You don't have to defend yourself. Instead of letting them get on your nerves, have some fun with them; quibble over absolute irrelevancies, throw back non sequiturs, recite nonsense poems, and confuse the heck out of them. As the saying goes, if you can't say anything nice, say something surreal.

If you're without kith or kin, or your family simply doesn't support you, seek support elsewhere. It's very important to find advocates on your behalf. (See Chapter 11 for info on how to structure support for yourself.) When possible, invite your supporters home to share meals and chat. Perhaps you can even host some meetings at your place.

Communication, which is key to so many things, has some basic elements.

Avoiding conflict

You shouldn't be afraid of conflict; it's unavoidable in any relationship. You need to figure out how to work through disputes in a healthy manner.

Avoiding those you don't care about is one thing. With those whose lives are closely intertwined with yours, however, it's reasonable to want to explain your side of the story. If you're unable to resolve differences, however, take these tips to task:

- ✔ **Let it slide.** The best you can do in such cases is to agree to disagree.

- ✔ **Choose your battles carefully.** Conserve your energy for getting well. The erratic blood sugar syndrome may have left you feeling out of control, scrambling to put the pieces of your life together.

- ✔ **Show consideration for others.** Showing consideration will help avoid misunderstandings or disagreements. In the case of social situations, such as dinner invitations, you can show consideration by alerting your host or hostess in advance. (This topic is covered in more detail in Chapter 16.)

One man's ham

Here's a prime example of just how emotional some people can get about food. This sidebar also provides a lesson in the critical importance of communication, particularly when you're dealing with a culture that's different than your own.

Katie, an American expatriate living in Tokyo, is a vegetarian who prefers to eat whole, natural, healthy foods. It's very difficult to find restaurants in Japan that serve vegetarian fare, so she compromises when eating out with people. One evening she went to a restaurant with a group of friends. She ordered a bowl of noodles that the waitress assured her didn't contain meat. When the noodles were brought to her table, however, they were swimming in greasy meat — too much for her to pick aside. She therefore reminded the waitress that she didn't eat meat and sent the bowl back to the kitchen. When the waitress brought back some more noodles, they were smothered with strips of ham. At that point, Katie and her friends left the restaurant without paying for their food, which they hadn't touched.

Being hungry and crabby (with their blood sugar plummeting, no doubt), they hurled insults at the restaurant staff before taking off. The incensed cook chased them down, grabbed the most defenseless-looking woman, and beat her down. The women called the police, who then forced them to pay for their meal. Why? According to the policeman, the restaurant had acted in good faith by serving them a vegetarian dish. Ham, he pointed out, is not meat. Food that is generally accepted as vegetarian in Japan differs from what Westerners regard as vegetarian.

When in doubt — particularly if you're surrounded by hostile people — don't press the issue. Nibble on your snack if you're hungry and don't waste time arguing.

Maintaining your boundaries

When the poet Robert Frost wrote that good walls make good neighbors, he was presenting sensible advice on living. By erecting a wall (literally as well as figuratively), you ensure that your neighbors respect your privacy and refrain from sticking their noses in your business. Just as a wall around your house protects you from prying eyes and trespassers, maintaining healthy emotional and mental boundaries prevents people from meddling in your affairs and keeps them from getting unwanted control of you.

Boundary violations occur when people

- Tell you what you ought to be feeling
- Tell you what you ought to eat (unless they're medical professionals)

- Tell you how to run your life
- Suggest that you have no right to feel the way you do
- Make you feel guilty for having needs
- Make you feel guilty for needing reasonable accommodations
- Wonder out loud why you're always this or that (sick or tired, for example)
- Put you down or insult you in any way

Notice all the "oughts"? They ought not tell you how to be! But you ought to definitely

- **Be honest with yourself.** It will help you know very clearly what you need and what is destructive.

- **Let others know when you reach your limits or they trespass on your boundaries.** Be confident when expressing your limits and boundaries.

- **Set very clear limits regarding what you will tolerate.** When others make demands on your time and energy that you can't comfortably honor because of your health issues, calmly tell them so (in no uncertain terms).

- **Offer choices when someone makes demands you can't honor comfortably.** One way to handle the demands of others is to give them a choice. For instance, you can say, "I can either take the kids to the ball game or cook dinner, but not both. Which do you want me to do?" Make sure that you provide a clear message that you want to do your share, but you can't be expected to do everything. You'll be leaving room to work out a compromise.

- **Watch your tone.** It's not so much what you say but how you say it. If you whine, people react negatively. If you sound uncertain, others question you. Be as confident and upbeat as you can. Make your requests sweet and simple. And smile.

Sabotaging the saboteurs

Your critics — inner and outer — try to sabotage your best efforts. You'll always find people who delight in criticizing you, tormenting you, and making you doubt that anything you do will ever improve your health. Or maybe they don't set out to destroy you but they whine about everything. Either way, these people are negative because they're unhappy with themselves.

Others

Like alcoholics who discover that they need a different circle of friends if they are to stay sober, you may have to let go of some friendships that are no longer serving your purpose. Bad friends prod you to go off your food program or complain that you're no longer any fun because you don't wash down a whole chocolate cake with root beer, or chug-a-lug a jug of beer as you scarf down mashed potatoes and deep-fried chicken.

Here are some suggestions for what to do when your critics start harping on about your new lifestyle, and no amount of reasoning on your part makes a dent. These suggestions are by no means a staple of good communication. But they sure can be fun!

- ✔ Walk out of the room.
- ✔ Interrupt them repeatedly.
- ✔ Laugh hysterically and don't explain why.
- ✔ Keep saying that you don't understand, and ask them to repeat themselves until you wear them down.
- ✔ Agree with them wholeheartedly and continue doing what you have to do.
- ✔ Thank them for sharing.
- ✔ Pretend that they're not there.
- ✔ Insist that health is now your new priority, and simply end the discussion.

Yourself

If you're your own personal saboteur, get guidance on positive self-talk or cognitive therapy. These days you can find numerous good books and audio programs that teach you how to change habitual, negative, fear-based thinking into "real-based" thinking. With this type of thinking, you don't repeat mindless positive affirmations. Rather, you use affirming but realistic statements to steer your behavior in a more productive direction.

Chapter 14

Suffering Along with Your Sweetie?

*I*f you're living with — or closely interacting with — a hypoglycemic, you know that it's not exactly what you'd call a Sunday picnic in the park. You may have discovered that your family member, aside from any admirable qualities he may possess, isn't exactly made of sugar, spice, and everything nice. He may be the sweetest, most charming, and most considerate person in the world one minute, purring along contentedly, and the next minute, he may suddenly turn his fangs on you. Indeed, you may wonder if your family member isn't suffering from a Jekyll-and-Hyde type personality. You're right, in a sense.

Depending on how severe the symptoms are, a hypoglycemic is probably taking quite a ride. He may be experiencing a roller coaster of chaotic emotions and unpredictable mood shifts. Life may have simply become unmanageable. If so, take heart. It can all be turned around. If your loved one follows the eating program outlined in this book, he or she will soon be restored to sanity. How soon he finds relief from his symptoms depends on various factors, such as age, body constitution, discipline, and so on. In most cases, though, some measure of relief is felt after several weeks; you should see major changes after several months.

And here's where you come into the picture. Whether you're the spouse, lover, parent, child, or friend of a hypoglycemic, your support can make all the difference in the world. You can offer up this support in several forms: Improving your knowledge about the disease, using productive communication, joining your love in the preparation of food, and improving your own eating habits can all help. You can make recovery from this pernicious condition faster, smoother, and easier.

Saying Hello to Mr. Hyde

So you've got a Hyde on your hands: Your loved one is lashing out, and you're bearing the brunt. You can run from Hyde (pun intended), or you can remember that Jekyll is in there. You're already solidly on the road to showing support: You're here, aren't you?

To offer the right kind of support, a solid understanding of hypoglycemia is useful. As with any illness, the more knowledge you have, the better. For starters, you can

- **Read this book.**
- **Check out other resources on hypoglycemia.** Chapter 17 lists Web sites and resources that provide information about hypoglycemia. You can also find many books on the subject at your local library or bookstore.
- **Talk to other hypoglycemics and their families.**
- **Consult with knowledgeable healthcare practitioners.**
- **Discuss the disorder with the sufferer.**

Pursuing these paths to knowledge can lead you directly into the gaping mouth of what you run up against during one of Hyde's horrible hissy fits: symptoms.

Recognizing the typical signs of low blood sugar is crucial to helping yourself and your loved one. Common symptoms (which are discussed in more detail in Chapter 3) include

- Irritation
- Mental confusion
- Temper outbursts
- Crying jags
- Forgetfulness
- Excessive yawning (despite adequate sleep)
- Suddenly and inexplicably falling asleep (even when not in bed!)

Macro Michio and the coffee conundrum

Followers of the macrobiotics diet (a natural health diet that originated in Japan) like to repeat the following story about Michio Kushi, one of the foremost leaders of the natural foods macrobiotics movement. One day Kushi and an acquaintance walked into a coffee shop to chat. They both ordered coffee, but Kushi left his untouched. When the acquaintance asked him about it, Kushi reportedly answered, "I've already paid for the coffee. Why should I pay for it twice?"

And pay for it you will if you have the sensitive biochemistry of a hypoglycemic. Although coffee is pleasantly stimulating and can uplift the spirit when consumed in moderation, it can also lead to a blood sugar crash and all its subsequent symptoms. (You can read more about the effects of caffeine in Chapter 2.)

The number, frequency, and severity of symptoms differ for each individual. Some people may only be mildly affected by symptoms, but it's probably fair to say that, for most hypoglycemics, life is a constant battle. They often struggle to get going and keep going when the spirit is willing but the body is flagging. Far too many have paid the price in checkered careers, strained interpersonal relationships, and unfulfilled dreams. And you, too, as a family member, have paid the price. Fortunately, you can do something about the symptoms associated with hypoglycemia.

Knowing what to expect can lead you to talk with your family member about what she is going through. As you discuss the ways that you can make it easier for her to change her diet and anything else that may be impeding her progress, your supporting role becomes more clear. The road to recovery starts with communication.

Talking It Over

Your loved one may act like a beast when she's having an attack of low blood sugar, but remember that she's a human being, and so are you. Use your tongue and teeth to talk to each other, not to tear each other to shreds. Words can heal as much as they can hurt; you just have to know the right words to say. When someone's acting out, knowing what to say and what not to say can help keep a volatile situation from getting out of control. It's an easy enough skill to develop, but because it's not something you're likely to know instinctively, we offer you the four Rs.

You can put the four Rs into action by following these steps:

1. **Recognize that when your loved one has hissy fits, it's the low blood sugar talking.**

   Don't take hypoglycemic symptoms personally. When a person has a hypoglycemic episode, not enough sugar is getting into the brain. The first area of the brain to shut down is the *neocortex* (the "civilized" portion of the brain), where higher learning and thinking take place. (Chapters 1 and 2 discuss this topic in greater detail.)

2. **Refrain from getting involved in the drama.**

   Avoid these things:

   - Criticizing

   - Reasoning with the person

   - Getting drawn into an argument

   Of course, it's all too human to react negatively if someone snaps at you or behaves in an inappropriate fashion. Delivering a comeback may feel most natural and satisfying in the heat of the moment, but you only end up frustrating yourself. Not only do you fail to accomplish anything but you may also make the battle escalate.

3. **Respond with compassion.**

   The following sections tell you how to convey your supportive feelings to the sufferer.

4. **Remind the hypoglycemic to eat.**

   Offer high-quality snacks. The snacks should have some protein and complex carbs: a boiled egg or a stick of celery with nut butter, for example. Do *not,* under any circumstances, provide anything with sugar and refined flours. You can rule out sodas, pastries, cookies, and ice cream, among other common snacks. (See Chapter 6 for acceptable snacks.) Remember that even a small amount of sugar or simple carbs can trigger symptoms.

You can always walk away from the situation for a while. After the dust settles and your loved one's blood sugar returns to normal (whatever her optimal level may be), she'll most likely apologize profusely. When the reconciliation begins, you can at last attempt to have a discussion. If you need to make a joint decision about something, this is the time to do it. Don't try to make important decisions when her brain has shut down from lack of fuel.

To help keep the dust down while your family member is calm, the following sections give you some general do's and don'ts for communicating with a hypoglycemic who's attempting to overhaul her diet and possibly change her exercise and work habits, as well.

Giving these words the green light

People are apt to think of low blood sugar sufferers as lazy and undisciplined, or as hypochondriacs who dream up imaginary illnesses in a desperate bid for attention. Low blood sugar sufferers receive little, if any, sympathy or understanding — even from themselves! They're often met with blame, criticism, or irritation.

Hypoglycemia is not all in the mind, however. Recognized or not, something is going on physiologically. Hypoglycemia isn't some unfortunate fad, such as a bad haircut or a fabricated disease de jour, that people choose so that they can stand apart from the crowd or gain sympathy. No wounds or scars may be visible, but the suffering is all too real.

Because hypoglycemia is a legitimate condition, the sufferer needs you to offer encouragement, sympathy, and support. You need to become an advocate, especially during hypoglycemic attacks, when the person is unable to think clearly. (These attacks are usually a result of forgetting to eat.) Again, remind yourself that it's the low blood sugar, not the sufferer, that's the problem. (See "Talking It Over," earlier in this chapter, for more tips on how to handle hypoglycemic attacks.)

When hypoglycemics feel discouraged, feel that they aren't healing fast enough, or feel that their diet isn't working, you can simply point out to them which symptoms have disappeared. Forgetting how things used to be is easy. Because most people have a tendency to concentrate on the negative — or on the symptoms that they continue to have — they may not notice that some of their symptoms have disappeared. Encourage your loved one to fill out the self-questionnaire in Chapter 4 if she hasn't already done so. Keep a copy of her completed questionnaire for yourself so that you can refer back to it from time to time and remind her of how she used to be (and of how far she has come).

The following list includes some words of encouragement you can give to someone who's working to control her hypoglycemia:

- ✔ "You're on the right track."
- ✔ "You're doing great."
- ✔ "I'm so proud of you."
- ✔ "You're so much better than you used to be."
- ✔ "I can really see a positive difference in you."
- ✔ "Remember how you used to be? You've come a long way (baby)."
- ✔ "Have you noticed that you're no longer suffering from [insert specific symptom here]?"

Putting the brakes on these words

One big drawback to suffering from hypoglycemia is that it's just not widely understood. It doesn't seem quite as legitimate as some of the more serious illnesses or disorders, such as cancer or diabetes, particularly because the medical profession generally doesn't recognize it. Lab tests, discussed in Chapter 5, can't always give a proper diagnosis of hypoglycemia. Because hypoglycemia has such a vast array of puzzling symptoms, it can feel like an anything-goes, catch-all syndrome — hardly something you can take seriously.

If you want to show that you care and you understand the full ramifications of low blood sugar, avoid these statements:

- ✔ "Snap out of it."
- ✔ "Grow up."
- ✔ "Get a life."
- ✔ "You're crazy."
- ✔ "It's all in your head."
- ✔ "What's your problem?"
- ✔ "Why can't you be like everyone else?"

Low blood sugar or not, it's best to refrain from negative comments, as they may make the other person defensive, leading them to shut down communication. Negative comments are definitely not for nurturing a relationship. But if you do slip up, don't be too hard on yourself. The vast majority hasn't achieved sainthood yet, so just apologize and let it go. Don't let yourself engage in an escalating battle of blame.

Keep in mind that making dietary and lifestyle changes is difficult. You're bound to experience plateaus and what may appear to be setbacks. Low blood sugar sufferers — who are probably prone to be sensitive anyway — may feel quite discouraged.

To get everyone in the family on the same page, you may consider calling a family meeting. Lay down some basic do's and don'ts, such as comments that should be avoided or things that family members can do to support the hypoglycemic person. Make sure that no one in the family makes comments such as these:

- "C'mon, one bite won't hurt you." (No, but it can trigger a full-blown binge.)

- "Just start the diet tomorrow." (And tomorrow, and tomorrow, and tomorrow . . .)

- "It's a holiday." (Or your birthday, or your anniversary, or the first day of the rest of your life. . . . The body doesn't care what occasion it is.)

- "What are you being so strict for? You don't need to lose weight." (The diet isn't about losing weight.)

- "You'll get sick if you don't eat." (Eating the wrong foods will make hypoglycemics sick, too.)

- "What a scrumptious dessert!" (It's nothing compared to the scrumptiously debilitating side effects the hypoglycemic will get from eating it.)

- "Don't tell me you're still trying to follow that crazy diet!" (What's crazy is the persistence of eating foods that cause havoc to the hypoglycemic's metabolism — not to mention his life.)

- "What are you, some kind of health nut?" (Would you say that to a diabetic who has to watch his diet?)

Offering Your Offspring Support

As a parent, it's up to you to figure out if your child is hypoglycemic. Because children can't be expected to fill out the self-questionnaire in Chapter 4, you should observe your child closely and answer the questions for her.

If your child is showing symptoms of low blood sugar (flip to Chapter 3 for a list of symptoms), consider taking her to the doctor. (Chapter 5 shows you how to find the right healthcare professional.) Don't assume that it's just a phase that she's going through and that she'll grow out of it. If you leave the dysfunction uncorrected, it's liable to get worse. Having low blood sugar in the formative years may be even more damaging than having it as an adult, as children are still learning important skills. Children may be sluggish or lack motivation to do well if their symptoms aren't taken care of.

If your child is hypoglycemic, don't make her feel isolated or different. Explain why she has to change her eating habits, and find healthy snacks that she can enjoy (see suggestions in Chapter 6). Find the time to bake some healthy desserts for her if at all possible. It can boost morale enormously if everyone in the family follows a (mostly) hypoglycemic diet. Hypoglycemic diets are actually very healthy for everyone, with only a few modifications required.

With children, you may need to provide even more encouragement to make sure that they follow the food plan. Getting them off sugar and junk food completely may be very difficult. You can help them by gradually changing their diet and offering them lots of love and positive talk. Never threaten or belittle them. Give them nonfood rewards for making the necessary changes. Make it okay to go off the food plan once in a while so that they don't feel too restricted.

Jumping In with Both Feet (and 2.5 Kids, a Dog, and a Cat)

The lifestyle changes recommended in this book can benefit anyone. Today, most everyone suffers from stress and requires some form of exercise, and no one can function forever without proper rest and relaxation. Having a low blood sugar sufferer in your family (or your circle of friends) may be just the wake-up call you need. Take this opportunity to review your life, your diet, and your priorities.

Turn the project of healing hypoglycemia into a family affair. Then, not only do you cement the bonds of your relationship but you also enable your loved one to recover much faster. For instance, assign one person to remind the resident hypoglycemic to eat every one-and-a-half to two hours. Here are some other tips that may help you get the whole family involved:

> ✔ **Talk openly if you have any reservations or concerns.** Do you feel threatened? Criticized? Made to feel wrong? Share your thoughts and feelings with your resident hypoglycemic

as well as with other low blood sugar sufferers and their families.

- ✔ **Turn the challenge of making dietary and lifestyle modifications into a game.** For instance, you can have a family brainstorm session to come up with ways to make reviewing and changing your lifestyle easier. Another idea is to have a drawing or lottery to determine who does the different cooking and household chores. Or whip up new recipes that fit into the food plan. Be creative! Even if you don't have kids, you can still have fun making these changes! If you do have kids, get them involved.

- ✔ **Show solidarity and support, but don't let the hypoglycemic act like a drama queen.** If she does flaunt an air of unspeakable sorrow, gently remind her that everyone has a cross to bear, but you're happy to help share some of the burden.

- ✔ **Don't make the journey back to health painful, solemn, or hard work.** Take it with humor, and take it as lightly as you can, but don't pull a long face and become morbidly serious.

Whether out of ignorance or fear, it's often family members who most resist change.

You Be Betty Crocker and I'll Be Julia Child

When you live with a hypoglycemic, mealtime can't be a slapdash affair where you veg out in front of the TV with a bag of chips in hand. Nor can you simply order a pizza (although you can make a

---

Easy does it

Hey, don't let the prospect of reviewing your lifestyle overwhelm you. Even small changes can work wonders. Just don't stress yourself out in a Herculean attempt to alter everything at once. Easy does it. Rather than thinking of lifestyle changes as more work and responsibility, consider ways to turn them into pleasure. For instance, you can have fun, spend time with your family, and engage in a good workout by enjoying some outdoor sports together, such as hiking and cycling. Or you can motivate both yourself and the person with hypoglycemia by buddying up with him or her and exercising together. (For more on exercise, see Chapter 8.) And whatever you do, have compassion, both for yourself and for the sufferer of low blood sugar.

healthy homemade version). Because eating junk food isn't a good idea, you have to put more thought into cooking and shopping for groceries.

After you create a routine, though, the meal preparations shouldn't take up too much more of your time. If everyone in the family chips in, your meals can be fun. The adults can take turns shopping and cooking, and the children — if you have children — can contribute according to their age and ability. Chapter 11 has great tips on how to make meals a nice part of your life together.

Make sure that you serve meals on a regular schedule! Remember, if your family member's blood sugar drops too low, you may have one easily angered person on hand.

As we mention earlier in this chapter, you're better off if everyone in the family converts to a more or less hypoglycemic diet. Changing your diet makes everything so much simpler — not to mention healthier! Of course, you don't have to eat as frequently as the hypoglycemic. You may want to stick to three average-size meals (not restaurant portions: too big!) and perhaps one snack. You most likely share just one meal a day with the resident hypoglycemic.

If you don't suffer from low blood sugar, you don't have to restrict your intake of carbs as much — you can consume 50 to 60 percent of your calories in the form of complex carbs. You can probably cut yourself more slack than the hypoglycemic, as you can eat off-limit foods on occasion. However, don't eat off-limit foods too often, and, if possible, try not to eat them in front of the hypoglycemic. Remember, tempt not, taunt not, flaunt not. Your loved one will appreciate your consideration, and you'll more likely enjoy peace of mind. Do unto others as you would have them do unto you. Changing your diet is hard enough without having temptation thrust in your face!

If you're adamant about sticking to your own diet, you can still eat part of your meals together. Everyone needs greens (lots of greens), so make them the dishes you both eat. Either the main dish or the side dish can be fixed separately. You may be able to cook most of the meal at the same time. For instance, if the main dish calls for sugar, you can set aside a portion with no added sugar for the hypoglycemic and then add the forbidden ingredient to the rest of the food. Use your creativity and ingenuity to find what works best for you.

Chapter 15

Relief at the Tip of Your Tongue

*A*ll the recipes in this chapter are acceptable for hypoglycemics. Many are quick and easy to fix — just what you need when you're too tired and you don't feel up to following complicated directions. You can mix and match as you like, but be sure to combine some protein, vegetables, starch, and fat with each meal.

Although alcohol is not recommended for hypoglycemics, it's generally okay to use small amounts of cooking wine. If you find that you have problems with wine, however, you can simply omit it.

Apple Banana Pancakes

Top these pancakes with fruit instead of maple syrup. Fruit can help you better control your blood glucose by limiting the amount of sugars you eat.

Preparation time: 15 minutes

Cooking time: 10 minutes

Yield: 4 servings (12 pancakes — 3 per person)

¾ cup all-purpose flour

½ cup whole wheat flour

2 teaspoons baking powder

¼ teaspoon salt

1½ teaspoons applesauce

2 teaspoons apple juice concentrate

1¼ cups lowfat milk

3 egg whites

2 overripe bananas, mashed well

Nonstick cooking spray

1 In a bowl, combine all-purpose flour, whole wheat flour, baking powder, and salt. Set aside.

2 In another bowl, combine applesauce, apple juice concentrate, milk, egg whites, and bananas. Stir well. Add flour mixture. Stir until smooth. (Pancake batter thickens as it sits. If you don't immediately cook the pancakes, or if the cooking extends over a period of time, you may need to thin the batter with a little more milk as you cook each batch.)

3 Coat a large, well-seasoned or nonstick skillet with cooking spray. Heat skillet over medium heat until hot. For each pancake, spoon ¼ cup of batter onto skillet. When bubbles form on top of pancakes, after about 1 to 1½ minutes, turn them over. Cook until bottom of each pancake is golden brown. Serve immediately, topped with fruit of your choice.

Nutrient analysis per serving: 245 kcalories, 10 grams protein, 49 grams carbohydrate, 1.6 grams fat, 0.7 grams saturated fat, 3 milligrams cholesterol, 4 grams fiber, 409 milligrams sodium

Exchanges: 3 starch

Breakfast Pizza

As any cook knows, eggs can be served in so many ways — incorporated into salads, added to sauces and meat loaf, and, as in this recipe, used as the filling for an inventive sandwich that was inspired by the pleasures of pizza. A small amount of shredded cheese is made to stretch, supplying plenty of flavor without all the calories of America's favorite fast food!

Preparation time: *15 minutes*

Cooking time: *20 minutes*

Yield: *4 servings*

1 loaf French or Italian bread	*⅛ teaspoon garlic powder*
Nonstick cooking spray	*⅛ teaspoon black pepper*
1 tablespoon unsalted butter	*4 whole eggs*
½ small onion, finely chopped	*8 egg whites*
4 medium red potatoes, boiled, diced small	*½ cup shredded reduced-fat cheddar cheese*

1 Preheat oven to 350 degrees Fahrenheit.

2 Cut bread in half lengthwise. Scoop out half of soft center. Place bread crust cut side up on a baking sheet coated with cooking spray, and spread bread with butter.

3 Coat a large, well-seasoned or nonstick skillet with cooking spray and place over medium heat. Sauté onions, stirring often, until tender, about 5 minutes. Spray the pan again with oil if necessary and add potatoes, garlic powder, and pepper. Sauté for 5 minutes.

4 In a bowl, whisk together eggs and egg whites. Add to onion-potato mixture. Cook over medium heat, stirring to scramble, until eggs are cooked.

5 Spoon egg mixture into bread. Sprinkle cheese on top. Bake 8 to 10 minutes until cheese melts. Cut each half of the bread in half again, crosswise. Serve immediately.

Nutrient analysis per serving: *447 kcalories, 25 grams protein, 58 grams carbohydrate, 13 grams fat, 5.5 grams saturated fat, 225 milligrams cholesterol, 4 grams fiber, 632 milligrams sodium*

Exchanges: *4 starch, ½ fat, 2 medium-fat meat*

Roasted Red Pepper Dip

Don't wait until you give a party to whip up some dip. This mix of red peppers makes a mouth-watering snack food. As the peppers roast and char, they develop wonderful flavor. Scoop out some dip with a slice of raw turnip, a cucumber spear, or any other vegetable: It's an easy way to increase your intake of vegetables.

Preparation time: *30 minutes*

Cooking time: *8 minutes (included in the preparation time)*

Yield: *4 servings (1½ cups)*

3 red peppers	*¼ cup nonfat plain yogurt*
Nonstick cooking spray	*⅛ teaspoon white pepper*
⅓ cup lowfat sour cream	*⅛ teaspoon salt*
⅓ cup nonfat mayonnaise	

1 Stem and seed the red peppers and then cut them in half lengthwise.

2 Use one of the following methods to cook the red peppers:

To oven-roast peppers: Preheat oven to 500 degrees Fahrenheit. Lightly coat the peppers with oil. Put them on a roasting pan and place the pan on an upper rack in the oven. Roast, shaking the pan occasionally, until peppers are browned and have collapsed, about 30 minutes. Proceed to Step 3.

To broil peppers: Preheat broiler. Lightly coat the peppers with oil. Place the peppers in a roasting pan and set it under the broiler, 3 to 4 inches from the heat. Broil, turning occasionally, until they are evenly browned and blistered, about 10 minutes. Some charring is fine, but don't let the peppers burn too badly. Proceed to Step 3.

To grill peppers: Preheat grill. Lightly coat the peppers with oil and place them on the grill. Cover and cook, turning occasionally, until the peppers are blistered and have collapsed, about 10 minutes. Some charring is fine, but don't let the peppers burn too badly. Proceed to Step 3.

3 Transfer the peppers to a bowl, cover tightly with foil or plastic wrap, and set aside until they're cool enough to handle. Peel the skin from the peppers.

4 Add red peppers, sour cream, mayonnaise, yogurt, pepper, and salt to a food processor and process until smooth.

5 Transfer dip to a bowl and then cover and chill.

6 Serve with fresh vegetables, such as broccoli florets, cauliflower florets, carrot sticks, celery sticks, cherry tomatoes, radishes, scallions, and zucchini.

Nutrient analysis per serving: 72 kcalories, 2 grams protein, 12 grams carbohydrate, 2.5 grams fat, 1.5 grams saturated fat, 8 milligrams cholesterol, 2 grams fiber, 252 milligrams sodium

Exchanges: 2 vegetable, 1 fat

Wild and Brown Rice Pilaf with Toasted Pecans

Try this pilaf made with brown rice and wild rice. The tawny flavor of toasted pecans is the perfect flavor complement to these whole grains. Nuts also increase the fat content of this dish, helping to balance the starchy carbohydrates of the grains.

Preparation time: 10 minutes

Cooking time: 45 minutes

Yield: 4 servings

1 orange, preferably organic

⅔ cup brown rice

⅓ cup wild rice

2½ cups lowfat chicken broth

¼ cup pecan halves

1 Using a zester, peel off small strips of orange peel. Place on a cutting surface and chop fine.

2 In a medium-size pot with a tightly fitting lid, combine the orange zest, brown rice, wild rice, and chicken broth. Bring to a boil over high heat and cover. Reduce heat to low and cook, covered, until tender and all of the liquid has been absorbed, about 45 minutes.

3 Cut the pecans lengthwise. Place a small sauté pan over medium-high heat and add the pecans. Heat the pecans, stirring constantly, until aromatic and slightly browned, about 2 minutes. Transfer to a small bowl and let cool to room temperature.

4 When the pilaf has finished cooking, add the pecans, toss, and serve immediately.

Nutrient analysis per serving: 230 kcalories, 6 grams protein, 40 grams carbohydrate, 5 grams fat, 0.5 grams saturated fat, 0 milligrams cholesterol, 3 grams fiber, 356 milligrams sodium

Exchanges: 2½ starch, ½ fat

Hearty Vegetable Soup

The U.S. Department of Agriculture's Dietary Guidelines for Americans suggests at least five servings of fruits and vegetables every day to ensure adequate intake of vitamins, minerals, and fiber. Enjoying a bowl of vegetable soup is a delicious way to meet your quota.

When you prepare this vegetable soup, first add the items that require longer cooking (such as beets or carrots), and then later add the quick-cooking ingredients (such as spinach and tomatoes). You'll have all your vegetables just where you want them (done to perfection) when your soup is finished. However, this procedure requires your time and attention. Another way to make sure that all the vegetables finish cooking at about the same time is to cut the longer-cooking types (such as potatoes) into smaller pieces, and the faster-cooking types (such as squash) into larger chunks.

Preparation time: *15 minutes*

Cooking time: *30 minutes*

Yield: *4 servings*

Nonstick cooking spray	*½ cup diced zucchini*
½ cup diced onions	*1 bay leaf*
½ cup diced celery	*⅛ teaspoon thyme*
½ cup diced carrots	*½ teaspoon oregano*
1 cup diced fresh yuca	*2 cups low-sodium chicken broth*
½ cup diced fresh tomatoes	*⅛ teaspoon white pepper*

1 Choose a large pot with a tightly fitting lid. Coat the pot with nonstick spray. Cook onion, celery, and carrots, stirring constantly, until onions are translucent — about 5 to 7 minutes. You can spray the pot with additional cooking spray or add a little stock or water if the vegetables begin to stick or burn. Add remaining ingredients and stir to combine.

2 Bring vegetable soup to a boil over high heat, uncovered, and then simmer covered for 20 minutes.

3 Serve immediately as a light lunch or mini meal.

Note: *Adding salt is optional, but it does increase the sodium level.*

Nutrient analysis per serving: *33 kcalories, 2 grams protein, 6 grams carbohydrate, 0 grams fat, 0 grams saturated fat, 0 milligrams cholesterol, 2 grams fiber, 212 milligrams sodium*

Exchanges: *½ starch*

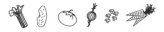

Oriental Beef and Noodle Salad

If you have a craving for Chinese takeout, satisfy your hunger with this healthy, lowfat salad, full of Asian flavor. Using a minimum of meat and lots of vegetables is typical for Chinese cooking. Although this style of cooking evolved by necessity (due to a scarcity of meat), the result of this hardship was the creation of an exceptionally healthy cuisine. This beef and noodle salad, made with lean meat and a minimum of cooking oil, is a good example of healthy Chinese cuisine.

Preparation time: *25 minutes*

Cooking time: *None*

Yield: *4 servings*

8 ounces thin spaghetti	¼ teaspoon ground ginger
4 teaspoons sesame oil	1 clove garlic, minced
Nonstick cooking spray	⅛ teaspoon white pepper
1 pound boneless top sirloin steak, trimmed of fat, cut 1 inch thick, and cut into slices about ¼-inch thick	2 tablespoons thinly sliced green onion
	2 tablespoons finely chopped red bell pepper
2 teaspoons low-sodium soy sauce	2 teaspoons chopped fresh cilantro
2 teaspoons red wine vinegar	
1 teaspoon Dijon mustard	

1 Bring a large pot of water to boil. Salt the boiling water and cook the spaghetti according to package directions, typically 5 to 6 minutes. Drain, rinse under cold running water, and drain again. Transfer to a large bowl and toss with the sesame oil, and then set aside.

2 Coat a large cast-iron or nonstick skillet with cooking spray and place over medium-high heat until hot. Add steak slices and cook until medium rare, about 1 minute per side. Add the steak to the bowl with the pasta.

3 In a small bowl, whisk together the soy sauce, vinegar, mustard, ginger, garlic, and white pepper. Add the green onions and red pepper and toss well. Add the mixture to the bowl with the spaghetti and steak and toss well.

4 Divide among four serving plates, sprinkle with cilantro, and serve.

Nutrient analysis per serving: *460 kcalories, 42 grams protein, 43 grams carbohydrate, 12 grams fat, 3 grams saturated fat, 82 milligrams cholesterol, 1.5 grams fiber, 180 milligrams sodium*

Exchanges: *4½ lean meat, 3 starch*

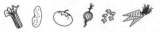

Spinach Pie

Who says you can't get a good vegetable into a delicious snack? You can fill an omelet with sautéed sweet peppers and onions, or grill tomatoes and onions to serve with smoked fish and breads the way the English do. A serving of this spinach pie has the further advantage of being low in fat.

Preparation time: *15 minutes*

Cooking time: *50 minutes*

Yield: *4 servings*

Nonstick cooking spray

1 package (10 ounces) frozen chopped spinach, thawed

1 medium yellow onion, thinly sliced

1 medium carrot, peeled and grated

1 cup low-sodium chicken broth

¼ teaspoon dried marjoram, crumbled

2 egg whites, lightly beaten

1 whole egg, lightly beaten

1 cup skim milk

1 cup shredded Swiss cheese

¼ teaspoon black pepper

1 Preheat oven to 350 degrees Fahrenheit.

2 Coat a 9-inch pie pan with nonstick cooking spray.

3 Squeeze all the water from spinach. Set aside.

4 In a small saucepan, cook onion and carrot with chicken broth and marjoram, uncovered, at low boil, stirring occasionally, until all liquid has evaporated and vegetables are nearly glazed, about 20 minutes. Spread vegetables out on a sheet pan to quickly cool.

5 In another bowl, whisk together egg whites and the whole egg. Add spinach, cooled onion, carrot, milk, cheese, and pepper.

6 Pour mixture into pie pan and bake uncovered, 25 to 30 minutes, until filling is set. Remove and cool.

Nutrient analysis per serving: *83 kcalories, 7 grams protein, 8 grams carbohydrate, 3 grams fat, 1 gram saturated fat, 7 milligrams cholesterol, 3 grams fiber, 129 milligrams sodium*

Exchanges: *3 vegetable, ¼ high-fat meat*

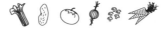

Apple Crisp

This lighter, healthier version of an old favorite is made without white sugar or fat. As a finale for dinner, have a little apple crisp to satisfy your sweet tooth, but because this dessert is full of carbohydrates, skip bread or other carbohydrate sources at this meal.

Preparation time: *25 to 30 minutes*

Cooking time: *50 to 55 minutes*

Yield: *8 servings*

3 large apples	*½ cup raisins*
½ cup rolled oats	*1 tablespoon lemon juice*
½ cup whole-wheat flour	*2 teaspoons cornstarch*
¼ cup Grape Nuts cereal	*2 tablespoons margarine, at room temperature*
1½ teaspoons cinnamon, divided use	
1 cup plus 3 tablespoons unsweetened apple juice, divided use	

1 Preheat oven to 350 degrees Fahrenheit. Spray or lightly grease a 9-inch pie dish.

2 Using a sharp paring knife, quarter the apples. Then, using a potato peeler or paring knife, peel the apples and cut out the core. Set aside.

3 *To make filling:* Whisk the cornstarch into a ¼ cup of the apple juice. In a large sauté pan, combine the apple juice–cornstarch mixture, ¾ cup of apple juice, the apples, raisins, ¾ teaspoon cinnamon, and lemon juice. Bring to a boil over high heat, and then reduce heat and simmer about 7 minutes, gently stirring occasionally to cook evenly. (Apples should be only slightly tender.) Remove apples and raisins with slotted spoon and place into the pie dish. Increase heat under sauté pan and maintain a low boil until sauce becomes syrupy. Pour sauce over apples and raisins.

4 *To make topping:* Combine rolled oats, whole-wheat flour, Grape Nuts, margarine, and ¾ teaspoon cinnamon in a medium bowl. Stir in up to 3 tablespoons of the apple juice, until the mixture holds together. Evenly dot over filling.

5 Bake for 30 minutes, until apples are bubbly and crust is lightly browned. Cool slightly and serve at room temperature or warm.

Nutrient analysis per serving: *226 kcalories, 3 grams protein, 46 grams carbohydrate, 5 grams fat, 0 grams saturated fat, 0 milligrams cholesterol, 5 grams fiber, 83 milligrams sodium*

Exchanges: *2 starch, 1 fruit*

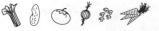

Black Bean Soup with Salsa Mexicana

A serving of this soup contains 43 grams of carbohydrate. But when you have a bowlful, only 33 grams of the total carbohydrates are available for your body to turn into glucose. The fiber in the beans reduces the effect carbohydrates have on your blood glucose.

Preparation time: 40 minutes

Cooking time: 3 hours

Yield: 8 servings

The Black Bean Soup

1 pound black beans

2 tablespoons vegetable oil

1 onion, chopped

1 small leek (white part only), chopped

4 cloves garlic, chopped

3 jalapeño chilies, seeded and membranes removed

½ bunch cilantro

1½ cups dark beer

1 quart chicken broth

1 quart water

1 smoked ham hock or smoked pork neck bones

½ teaspoon salt

Juice of 1 lime

The Salsa Mexicana

1 tablespoon minced garlic

3 tablespoons minced jalapeño

⅓ cup minced onion

⅓ cup red tomato, diced

⅓ cup yellow tomato, diced

2 tablespoons chopped cilantro

3 tablespoons fresh lime juice

1 tablespoon extra-virgin olive oil

1 Rinse the beans. Remove any stones and shriveled beans. Soak beans in enough cold water to cover them for 8 hours or overnight. Drain.

2 Heat the vegetable oil in a large pot over medium heat. Add the onions and leeks, and then sauté, stirring until soft, about 4 minutes. Stir in the garlic and jalapeños and cook for another minute. Add the drained beans, cilantro, beer, chicken stock, water, and ham hocks or neck bones. Bring to a boil. Lower heat and simmer, stirring occasionally, until the beans are very soft, about 2 hours. Skim off any foam that rises to the surface.

3 While the beans cook, prepare the Salsa Mexicana. In a medium bowl, combine the garlic, jalapeño, onion, red and yellow tomatoes, cilantro, lime juice, and olive oil, adding salt to taste (see the following note).

4 When the beans are soft, remove the ham hock or neck bones. Pour the beans into a blender or food processor, dividing into batches if necessary, and blend until smooth. Season to taste with salt and lime juice. The soup should be fairly thick but pourable. If soup is too thick, thin with additional hot chicken stock or water.

5 Serve soup in warm bowls garnished with Salsa Mexicana.

Note: *If you're on a low-salt diet, omit this added salt. This soup will still have enough salt, thanks to the salty ham hock.*

Nutrient analysis per serving: *313 kcalories, 16 grams protein, 43 grams carbohydrate, 8 grams fat, 1 gram saturated fat, 7 milligrams cholesterol, 10 grams fiber, 660 milligrams sodium*

Exchanges: *3 bread/starch, 1 lean meat*

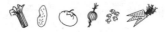

Cold Poached Salmon with Fresh Fruit Chutney and Herb Sauce

This recipe is great for company, because it can be prepared ahead of time — and you can rest assured that the fish will be moist. Just follow the instructions to cool the cooked salmon in its poaching liquid.

Preparation time: *40 minutes*

Cooking time: *5 to 8 minutes*

Yield: *4 servings*

4 cups water

6 tablespoons red vinegar

½ onion, thinly sliced

1 carrot, sliced

1 bay leaf

10 white peppercorns

1 to 2 teaspoons salt

4 pieces salmon fillet, 4 ounces each

The chutney:

1 papaya, peeled and diced finely

1 mango, peeled and diced finely

1 apple, peeled and diced finely

½ small red onion, diced finely

1 bunch cilantro, chopped

1 tablespoon crystallized ginger, minced

Juice from 1 lime

The herb sauce:

1 bunch spinach (about 10 ounces), tough stems removed

1 bunch tarragon or 1 teaspoon dried tarragon

1 bunch parsley, stems removed

1 bunch chives

1 clove garlic

1 cup light sour cream

1 tablespoon Worcestershire sauce

1 Bring the water to a boil in a large skillet and add vinegar, sliced onion, carrot, bay leaf, peppercorns, and salt. Add the salmon fillets, cover, and simmer 2 to 3 minutes. Remove from heat and let the salmon cool in the liquid in the skillet at room temperature.

2 *For the chutney:* Combine the papaya, mango, apple, onion, cilantro, lime juice, and ginger. Mix well; cover and let sit for 2 hours at room temperature or refrigerate if it needs to sit longer.

3 *For the herb sauce:* Bring 3 quarts of salted water to a rolling boil. Blanch the spinach and all herbs for 5 seconds. Drain. Put in blender or food processor with garlic and mince finely. Add sour cream and Worcestershire sauce and purée until smooth. Portion size is 2 tablespoons. Refrigerate unused sauce in a sealed container.

4 Place salmon fillets on individual plates, with a dollop of herb sauce and a spoonful of chutney next to the fish.

Nutrient analysis per serving: 278 kcalories, 29 grams protein, 29 grams carbohydrate, 6 grams fat, 2 grams saturated fat, 42 milligrams cholesterol, 6 grams fiber, 304 milligrams sodium.

Exchanges: 4 very lean meat, 2 fruit

Cowboy Shrimp with Jalapeño Cornsticks

This recipe offers a novel way of preparing shrimp that keeps its fat content low and adds some fiber from beans. One serving of this recipe provides almost half the recommended daily allowance of sodium. If you are restricting your intake of sodium, substitute toast or bread for the cornsticks, use low-sodium cheese and chicken stock, and avoid adding extra salt for flavoring. If using canned pinto beans, rinse to remove some of the sodium. And please note that you need cornstick molds to make this recipe.

Preparation time: *1½ hours*

Cooking time: *25 minutes*

Yield: *4 servings*

The shrimp:

¼ cup raw bacon, diced

½ cup onion, diced

3 tablespoons garlic, minced

3 tablespoons jalapeño, minced

1 tablespoon ground cumin

¼ cup tomato, diced

1 cup pinto beans, cooked

1 cup chicken stock or low-sodium chicken broth

12 large shrimp (10 to 15 shrimp per pound), peeled and deveined

Optional salt to taste

1 tablespoon olive oil

2 tablespoons fresh thyme, chopped

2 tablespoons cilantro, chopped

Lime juice to taste

2 ounces Queso Cotija, crumbled

Cilantro sprigs for garnish (optional)

The cornsticks:

Yield: *8 sticks*

1 cup cornmeal

1 cup flour

1 tablespoon baking powder

1 teaspoon salt (optional)

½ cup buttermilk

½ cup corn purée, cooked (can substitute an 8-ounce can of creamed corn)

3 tablespoons vegetable oil

2 or 3 jalapeños, seeded and minced

1 Heat heavy-bottomed saucepan over medium heat until hot. Cook bacon until crisp, about 3 to 5 minutes.

2 Drain fat, reserving 1 teaspoon. Add onions and garlic to the reserved fat. Cook 2 minutes.

3 Add jalapeño and cumin, sauté 1 minute, and then add tomato, pinto beans, and chicken stock. Simmer for 10 to 15 minutes.

4 Heat 1 tablespoon olive oil in a nonstick sauté pan until it is almost smoking. Sear shrimp until slightly browned, about 1 minute per side.

5 Add chopped thyme and cilantro. Cook until shrimp are just done, about another 1 to 2 minutes. Season with lime juice.

6 Preheat oven to 450 degrees Fahrenheit.

7 Place cornstick molds in oven until hot.

8 In a large bowl, combine cornmeal, flour, baking powder, and salt.

9 In separate bowl, beat together the buttermilk, corn purée, oil, and jalapeños. Add to the dry ingredients and mix until just combined.

10 Spoon the mixture into the cornstick molds and bake 10 to 12 minutes, until lightly browned (a toothpick inserted in the center should come out clean).

11 To serve, place one jalapeño cornstick on plate. Spoon pinto-bean mixture onto plate and over cornstick. Lay three shrimp on bean mixture, propped against cornstick. Sprinkle with Queso Cotija and garnish with cilantro sprig, if using.

Nutrient analysis per serving: 484 kcalories, 38 grams protein, 46 grams carbohydrate, 18 grams fat, 2 grams saturated fat, 189 milligrams cholesterol, 7 grams fiber, 950 milligrams sodium

Exchanges: 4 very lean meat, 3 starch, 2 fat

Loin of Pork Glazed with Roasted Vegetable Salsa

Loin of pork is preferred for oven-roasting, because slicing it for serving is so easy. However, loin of pork can easily become dry. This recipe specifies loin of pork with the bone left in, which yields moister, more flavorful meat and gives you more flexibility in timing.

Preparation time: *15 minutes*

Cooking time: *1½ to 2 hours*

Yield: *6 servings or more*

1 3- to 4-pound pork loin roast, bone-in

⅓ cup Roasted Vegetable Salsa

⅓ cup Dijon-style mustard

2 cloves garlic, minced

2 teaspoons minced fresh sage leaves or 1 teaspoon dried sage

½ teaspoon sea salt and freshly ground black pepper to taste

2 pounds potatoes, peeled and cut into 1-inch cubes

2 tablespoons olive oil, plus more as needed

1 Preheat the oven to 450 degrees Fahrenheit.

2 In a small bowl, mix together the garlic, sage, salt, and pepper.

3 Arrange the potatoes in a roasting pan that is also large enough to hold the pork. Toss the potatoes with 1 teaspoon of the garlic-sage mixture and olive oil. Place pan in the heated oven while you prepare the pork.

4 In a bowl, combine Roasted Vegetable Salsa and mustard. Spread the mixture over the pork.

5 Take the potatoes out of the oven, place the pork loin on top of the potatoes or alongside them, and put the pan back in the oven. Roast undisturbed for 30 minutes.

6 Remove roasting pan from the oven. Stir potatoes, using a spatula to scrape them off the bottom of the pan if necessary. Lower the heat to 325 degrees Fahrenheit and continue to cook, stirring the potatoes every 15 minutes or so.

7 After 1¼ hours total cooking time, check pork for doneness by inserting an instant-read thermometer into several places in the meat. When the thermometer reads 145 degrees Fahrenheit, remove roasting pan from the oven. Transfer the pork to a platter and let it rest for 10 to 15 minutes before carving. During the resting time, the temperature should continue to rise to 155 degrees Fahrenheit, leaving only a trace of rosiness in the center of the meat. (Cook pork to an internal temperature of 150 degrees Fahrenheit and a resting temperature of 160 degrees Fahrenheit if you prefer pork well done.)

8 Return the potatoes to the oven to keep warm, lowering the heat to 325 degrees Fahrenheit.

9 Carve the meat and serve the potatoes. Enjoy with a green vegetable such as sautéed zucchini. Savor the pork the next day in a sandwich, along with sautéed onions and more salsa.

Roasted Vegetable Salsa

Preparation time: *30 minutes*

Cooking time: *20 minutes*

Yield: *2½ cups*

1 pound ripe tomatoes	*½ cup tomato puree*
2 medium poblano chilies	*2 tablespoons chopped fresh cilantro*
2 red onions, sliced ¼-inch thick	*2 teaspoons fresh thyme leaves*
4 garlic cloves, peeled	*½ teaspoon salt*
2 teaspoons extra-virgin olive oil	*2 teaspoons cider vinegar*

1 Place tomatoes and chilies over the hot fire of a grill or in a broiler pan, and grill or broil on all sides until they are charred and blackened. Remove from grill or broiler and transfer to a large bowl. Loosely cover and set aside.

2 Heat oven to 425 degrees Fahrenheit.

3 Drizzle onions and garlic with 2 teaspoons olive oil. Toss them together to coat and then spread them in one layer on a baking sheet. Roast, stirring occasionally, until the onions are soft and brown and the garlic is soft and lightly browned in spots, about 15 minutes. Remove and cool at room temperature.

4 Peel the charred tomatoes and remove cores, catching any juice in a bowl. Add the peeled, cored tomatoes to the juice. Set aside. Peel chilies, remove seeds and stems, and cut into ¼-inch dice. Place chilies in a medium-size bowl.

5 Place roasted onion and garlic in a food processor fitted with a metal blade, and process until moderately finely chopped. Add to the bowl with the diced chilies and stir. Put the grilled tomatoes in the processor and process coarsely. Add chopped tomatoes, tomato puree, cilantro, and thyme to the bowl.

6 Season tomato salsa with salt. Stir in vinegar. Cover and refrigerate for a couple of hours to allow flavors to develop. Taste again before using and adjust flavors.

Nutrient analysis per 4-ounce serving: 398 kcalories, 36 grams protein, 26 grams carbohydrate, 16 grams fat, 4 grams saturated fat, 90 milligrams cholesterol, 3 grams fiber, 384 milligrams sodium

Exchanges: 4 lean meat, 2 starch, 1 fat

Roast Chicken with Red Onions and Potatoes

This beautiful and decorative platter is an eye-opener! The chicken goes very well with condiments like flavored mustards, pickles, and hot sauces. The red potatoes used in this recipe have a lower starch content than long white and russet potatoes.

Preparation time: 35 minutes

Cooking time: 75 minutes

Yield: 4 servings

2 3-pound chickens

3 tablespoons olive oil

1 tablespoon Dijon mustard

1 teaspoon fresh chopped thyme

1 teaspoon fresh chopped rosemary

½ teaspoon salt and pepper to taste

1 lemon, cut in half

4 medium red onions

8 round red potatoes

4 fresh thyme sprigs

4 fresh rosemary sprigs

1 Preheat oven to 350 degrees Fahrenheit.

2 Wash chickens under cold water. Using dry paper towels or a clean dishcloth, dry them off, and place in a large roasting pan.

3 Mix together oil and mustard. Rub chickens with this mixture. Sprinkle thyme, rosemary, salt, and pepper over the chickens. Squeeze 1 lemon half over the chickens. Cut the squeezed lemon half in two and place these in the cavity of each chicken. Reserve the other lemon half.

4 Peel the onions and cut them into large, thick rounds (about 4 slices per onion). Season with salt and pepper and put them into the pan with the chickens.

5 Wash potatoes and dry them. Rub them with olive oil, salt, and pepper, and put them into the pan along with the chickens and onions.

6 Place the roasting pan in the oven and cook until the chickens are done and the potatoes and onions are tender, about 1½ hours. They should finish cooking at the same time. Before removing the chickens from the pan, gently lift one side, tilting to let the juices run out of the cavity. If juice is red, cook another 5 minutes. A thermometer inserted in the thickest part of the thigh should read 160 to 165 degrees Fahrenheit.

7 Allow the chicken to rest for at least 8 minutes before cutting up and slicing. Cut the breast meat off the bone and detach the legs from the carcass. Arrange the chicken on a large serving platter and place the roasted onions and potatoes around it. Squeeze the other half of the lemon over the chicken and garnish with fresh thyme and rosemary sprigs.

Nutrient analysis per serving: 712 kcalories, 64 grams protein, 60 grams carbohydrate, 23 grams fat, 5 grams saturated fat, 180 milligrams cholesterol, 6 grams fiber, 478 milligrams sodium

Exchanges: 4 starch, 7 lean meat

Part VI
The Part of Tens

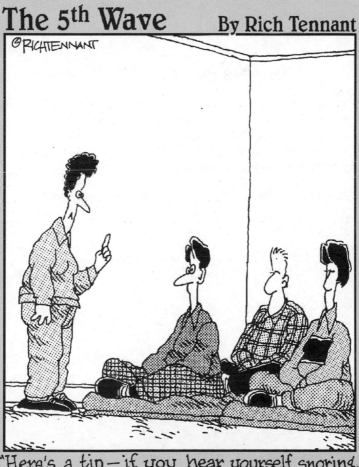

The 5th Wave   By Rich Tennant

@RICHTENNANT

"Here's a tip — if you hear yourself snoring, you're meditating too deeply."

In this part...

In this part, you find out what to do when temptation strikes. You discover how to better regulate your blood sugar, and you figure out what to do when you hit a snag. We provide you with ten tactics for staying on your food program, and ten hints for helping you deal with your condition. Finally, we refer you to helpful Web sites and other resources that can help you manage your own health.

Chapter 16

Ten Hints for Helping Hypoglycemics

● ●

In This Chapter
▶ Making changes to your diet and lifestyle
▶ Improving the performance of your brain

● ●

Maybe you're feeling like a sourpuss because, when it comes to hypoglycemia, there's so much to be careful about. It may seem daunting, but it's nothing you can't handle. You'll see for yourself that "doing" is indeed easier than "thinking about doing." With the tips compiled in this chapter, you won't have to be hyper-vigilant about your hypogylcemia. Besides, most of the dietary and lifestyle changes are good for you regardless of whether you have hypoglycemia.

Acting Practically at Home

Okay, so you have to work, eat, sleep, pay bills, do the laundry, and spend some quality time with those you love. Try to incorporate these things in what free time you have:

✔ Keep a list of foods to eat and foods to avoid on the fridge, and carry a copy with you wherever you go so that you can refer to it often. Chapter 6 gives further food fodder.

✔ Be prepared for emergencies. Don't go anywhere without food. Keep utensils, paper towels, and several coolers in your car, or bring a tote bag with snacks if you don't drive. Keep the coolers supplied with several days worth of food when you go on road trips.

> ✔ Review your food journal every week and make any necessary adjustments to your food plan. (Chapter 6 gives information on journaling.)
>
> ✔ Ventilate your house. If the air in your house is stagnant, stir it up with electric fans. You may also want to install an attic fan. Avoid using air fresheners.

Testing for Sugar

To eat or not to eat? Ah, what a dilemma! When eating out, you can't always tell whether a dish has sugar; the waitperson may not know, either.

Diabetes expert Dr. Richard Bernstein recommends carrying some Clinistix or Diastix (available at most pharmacies) to detect the presence of sugar or flour in packaged or restaurant foods. They're actually marketed for testing urine — but not to fear, he's not asking you to pee right at the table. To use these test strips for testing food, follow these steps:

1. **Put a small amount of food in your mouth.**

2. **Swish it or chew it around a bit so that it mixes with your saliva.**

3. **Spit a tiny bit onto a test strip.**

   The strip will change color if your food contains sugar. The darker the color, the more sugar it contains. The test strips will work on nearly all foods except milk products, which contain lactose. They also won't react with fructose.

Your family and friends are probably so used to your strange rituals involving food, that they probably won't even blink when you conduct this test. But if you're dining with business associates, you may want to perform the test in the bathroom or just skip it altogether and order only tried and true dishes. Grilled or broiled meat and fish are safe bets. You can order some steamed vegetables, or you can have salad with oil and vinegar (because most dressings contain sugar). If you can't have vinegar, sprinkle some lemon juice and a dash of salt on your salad.

Controlling Blood Sugar

Diabetics use glucose tablets to raise their blood sugar, but some low blood sugar sufferers report that glucose tabs help them, too.

Use glucose tabs with discretion. Taking them may put you in danger of a rebound drop in blood sugar. In other words, your body may produce too much insulin in response to the sugar, which in turn can cause your blood sugar to fall too low. Carry the tabs around with you in case of emergencies and use them only

- ✔ When you have very severe symptoms
- ✔ If you eat some protein within 20 minutes of taking them

Because glucose doesn't have to be digested, the tablets can raise your blood sugar rapidly with a predictable outcome. Dr. Richard Bernstein recommends Dextrotabs because they're inexpensive, conveniently packaged, and very easy to chew. Dextrotabs begin raising your blood sugar in about 3 minutes and stop raising it after about 40 minutes.

One point to bear in mind is that even if your blood sugar isn't too low, you may still have symptoms of hypoglycemia, such as a rapid heart rate, anxiety, tremors, and so on. If you wait a bit, they should abate.

Refrain from consuming too much during meals or snacks to avoid triggering too large an insulin response, which plays havoc with your blood sugar regulation. If you often feel hungry even after a reasonable meal, try finishing your meal with something that contains fat, as it tends to satisfy your appetite more. You may have a few slices of avocado or salad with lots of dressing. Also, if you're constantly hungry, you may not be getting enough of the right nutrients. You shouldn't get so hungry if you're eating frequent snacks. Review your diet and take some vitamins. (Check out Chapters 6 and 7 for more on diet and vitamins.)

Dos and Don'ts of Dining Out

Who doesn't eat out once in a while? Eating at a restaurant or a friend's home doesn't need to spell disaster. While you can't have your cake and eat it too (no cakes allowed on the food plan, unless it's homemade without sugar or refined flour), you can follow some simple guidelines to help manage your diet.

- ✔ About half an hour before going to a restaurant, eat a light snack. You never know how long you'll have to wait for a table or your order.
- ✔ Tell the waitperson about your allergies, sensitivities, and dietary restrictions, and don't be afraid to request modifications.

✔ Stay away from white rice, white bread, noodles, anything with sauces, chips, bean paste, barbecued meats, sweet and sour foods, meatloaf (it often contains sugar or sweetener), casseroles (no telling what ingredients are in them), and anything deep fried. (More on this in Chapter 6.)

✔ Because you're now eating smaller meals, most restaurant servings will be too large. To prevent overeating, measure out the amount you're going to eat and put the rest away in a doggie bag. Most restaurants in the United States serve such humongous portions that you can easily get three meals out of a single entrée. Think of all the money you're saving!

✔ Try ordering several appetizers instead of an entrée. It's a fun way to create a balanced meal. When ordering soups, be aware that they may be loaded with sugar.

✔ When your friends invite you to dinner, make your restrictions known but be gracious about it. Don't insist that they accommodate you.

   • Offer to bring a dish to share — something you can definitely eat.

   • Refuse politely when your host or hostess urges you to eat something you can't.

   • Don't be uncertain or apologetic.

   • Don't moan about your food restrictions, or your host may feel compelled to talk you into eating things that are off-limits.

✔ If everyone's having dessert and you're tempted beyond reason, order a sweet fruit (or bring some with you).

   • Although fruit juice isn't usually recommended, it's preferable to gooey desserts. (Drinking it at the end of a meal shouldn't cause too rapid a rise in blood sugar.)

   • If it's winter and you're cold, get a cup of tea and sweeten it with stevia, a natural low-carbohydrate sweetener. Carry several packets with you.

   • If all else fails, and you have to have a "real" dessert, get a bite from someone or share an order.

✔ You may find that there are times, such as special occasions, when you just have to have forbidden foods. In this case, you can go off your program, but make sure that you

   • Plan ahead — and be willing to pay the consequences.

   • Don't go off your program at a stressful time in your life — stress can aggravate hypoglycemia.

- Don't go off your program for too long.

- Always eat some protein to offset any sugar and concentrated carbs that you may eat.

✔ When staying with friends or relatives over a period of time, you may be able to make special requests if you have a close enough relationship with them. Otherwise, do what you can without imposing. Chapter 6 tells you more about diet, and Chapters 13 and 14 tell you how to live with a hypoglycemic. No matter what, be a considerate, gracious guest.

Food Facts for Tasty Health

They say that good medicine is bitter, but that's not always the case. Research is turning up more hard-core data about just how good certain foods (of course, we're talking natural stuff, like veggies and fruits, not prepackaged edibles) can be for your mind and body. In some cases, food can work like medicine — and it's probably the best-tasting medicine there is! The following facts about food can help you create a healthier diet:

✔ Unless you're cooking for an army, get smaller bottles of cooking oil. Add a capsule of vitamin E to the oil to help prevent oxidation, and throw out any oil that's been sitting for more than four months.

✔ It's preferable to use potato flour, barley flour, arrowroot flour, oat flour, or rice flour for thickening (replacing cornstarch).

✔ Milled flaxseed is one food you should definitely add to your diet. It promotes healthy sugar metabolism by slowing down sugar absorption. Its high fiber content helps keep you regular. It's also a boon to anyone at risk for type 2 diabetes. On top of that, it supports your immune system.

✔ To remove some of the starch from potatoes, cut them up and soak them in water overnight, and then drain them. To remove some starch from your oatmeal, cook it in twice the amount of water required, and then pour it through a strainer.

✔ You know what they say about eating an apple a day. Anyone with a blood sugar disorder should heed this advice. Apples and onions are rich in *quercetin* (a *flavonoid,* potent antioxidants found in most plants), which lowers the risk for developing type 2 diabetes, stroke, lung cancer, heart disease, and asthma.

✔ Fruits are good for you. The darkest fruits, such as black or red grapes, are the richest in antioxidants, which help detoxify the body.

✔ Almonds and turkey not only provide protein but they're also excellent sources of vitamin B6, which plays an important role in the synthesis of *serotonin* (the neurotransmitter that makes you feel calmer and happier).

✔ Toasted nori (seaweed), which is available in Asian markets, is high in nutrients and very low in calories. It's also good for sluggish thyroids. Eating kelp and seaweed daily for at least a month will help regulate your thyroid.

✔ Add protein shake powder to plain, full-fat yogurt, and sweeten with stevia. Or mix fruit-sweetened jam with some creamed cottage cheese. Be sure to get yogurt and cottage cheese with active cultures, as they may help grow beneficial bacteria in your intestines.

Noshing on Nourishment: Veggies and Nuts Do It Better

Vegetables make excellent nutrient-packed snacks. Make sure that you have a good supply of raw vegetables, such as broccoli, cauliflower, cucumbers, celery, and bell peppers, washed and cut into finger-sized pieces. For added flavor, dip them in red or white miso paste, or drizzle a little bit of salad dressing on them. Or try spreading nut butter, such as almond or cashew, on the vegetables. Some vegetables that you may want to try are

✔ **Leafy vegetables (such as kale or collards):** These vegetables can be cooked very quickly. Put them in a pot with just enough water to cover them. Boil for 3 or 4 minutes. Drain and freeze individual portions in baggies.

✔ **Salted green soybeans (edamame):** They're usually found frozen in Asian super markets. Cook them in boiling water for five minutes and drain. Cool them under running water before eating, or refrigerate and serve chilled.

✔ **Artichokes:** Steam or boil for about 45 minutes. You may want to try them with low-fat salsa or other dips you enjoy.

✔ **Steamed Brussels sprouts:** Like other members of the cruciferous family (like broccoli), they're thought to fight cancer. You can also boil them, covered, for 8 to 10 minutes, until they're slightly tender but still crisp. Keep individual portions of leafy green salads (also rich in vitamin E) in the fridge for snacking. Don't add the salad dressing until just before you eat.

- ✔ **Almonds and avocados:** They have vitamins that play an important role in the synthesis of serotonin, the neurotransmitter that helps you feel happy. Other good serotonin-boosters are tomatoes, eggplants, and walnuts.

- ✔ **Raw walnuts and pumpkin seeds:** These are great sources of Omega-3 fatty acids, which the modern diet tends to be low in. If you get tired of eating plain, raw pumpkin seeds, try Pumpkorn (seasoned pumpkin seeds), which can be found in natural food stores.

Brainy Foods

Did you know that the brain is made up of 60 percent fat? No kidding! If that was your body fat percentage, you'd be considered obese! The following nutrients can help your gray matter:

- ✔ **Vitamin E:** The brain is susceptible to harmful *oxidation* (a process that damages cells and genes). Taking plenty of vitamin E helps slow down oxidation and reduce memory loss. Brussels sprouts and avocados are good sources of vitamin E.

- ✔ **Omega-3 fatty acids:** This is found in fatty fish such as salmon, sardines, herring, mackerel, and anchovies. It helps your body to build more brain cells. Eating fish three to four times a week not only boosts your brain power but also lifts your mood. If you're a vegan, take one or two teaspoons of flax oil five times a week. Flax oil is also rich in Omega-3, so use it instead of butter on your bread, or add it to your salad.

- ✔ **Folate:** Legumes and green vegetables hold lots of folate, which is a B vitamin. All the B vitamins are very important in brain development and cognitive health.

Banishing Brain Fog

Uh, oh. The fog that just rolled in isn't outside the window. It's in your head. And the worst part is that because you can't think clearly, you can't quite figure out what to do. Fortunately, you can take action to alleviate the problem. Try the following suggestions and see if one, or a combination of them, works for you.

- ✔ **Chew gum.** Chewing gum may stimulate and improve your short-term memory. Studies have shown that there is an increase in the activity of the *hippocampus* (the area of the brain where new memories are stored) when people chew gum.

✓ **Use ozone air-purification machines regularly.** They're a boon to people who live or work in places with airborne pollutants, fumes, mold, mildew, and so on. You can get a portable machine for home use. You'll start to notice the benefits after two to three weeks.

✓ **Eat nutritious foods.** Nutritious foods not only enhance your memory and learning but they may also help dispel brain fog.

✓ **Kick caffeine.** It gives you a temporary buzz, but in the long-run, it aggravates your health condition. Instead of drinking coffee, you may want to try drinking the South American herb yerba mate, which can energize you and give you a lift without the coffee jitters.

✓ **Take oral DHEA (dehydroepiandrosterone).** DHEA is a steroid hormone. The concentration of DHEA in the human body plummets as people age. Studies suggest that DHEA improves memory and increases physical and psychological well-being. A daily dose of 30 to 90 mg may enhance the brain's ability to process and store information.

✓ **Shake, shake, shake your bod.** Let all your limbs go loose and roll your head freely while breathing naturally. Do it for anywhere from one to five minutes. It's an old Qigong exercise that helps you relax and sweep away any cobwebs from your mind. (Chapter 8 talks more about Qigong.) Here's another exercise you can try:

1. Stand with your knees slightly bent and your feet shoulder-width apart.

2. Bring your arms up, as if carrying a ball. Your elbows should be rounded, and your palms should face you. Your right and left fingertips should almost touch.

3. Close your eyes and take a few deep breaths. Imagine that you're standing in a waterfall. Water is running down your head, face, and body, clearing your mind and cleaning your body.

4. Do this exercise for five minutes to an hour.

✓ **Exercise your hands.** One exercise you can try is "dry washing." All you have to do is wring your hands, as though you're washing them, for one to five minutes. You can also hold golf balls in your palms and then roll them with your fingers; or you can just go through the motions empty-handed.

✓ **Give yourself a pat on the face.** Here's an exercise adapted from the Luohan Patting System of Yin Style Bagua (a school of Chinese martial arts and healing). Don't hit yourself too hard! You don't need to use a lot of force, just make it rhythmical.

1. Using cupped palms, slap your head from the front to the back, and to the sides above your ears.

2. Lightly strike your forehead, temples, and cheeks.

3. Count 1-2-3, 1-2-3, 1-2-3-4, 1-2-3, and then pause slightly before repeating the sequence. (Or you can repeat, "Hot cross buns, hot cross buns, 1-2-3-4, hot cross buns.")

✔ **Laugh!** Laughing out loud releases endorphins in the brain, which makes you more alert and clears that foggy feeling from your head. You don't actually have to have anything to laugh about. Going through the motions of laughing can also provide you with the same benefits.

Easily Remembered Solutions to Short-Term Memory Loss

The brain has a higher metabolic rate than other organs, so if it isn't getting enough oxygen, glucose, and other substances that the brain cells need to function, your thinking may get fuzzy. You may find yourself spending several hours every day looking for misplaced items or forgetting things that should be second nature to you, such as remembering to take your wallet with you.

The best way to deal with this short-term memory loss is to

✔ **Write down everything that's important.** Keep a written record for everything, such as credit card payments, health care information, and so on.

✔ **Put lists everywhere.** Make sure that you place them someplace visible. Write appointments, messages, and reminders on a wall calendar and a day planner.

✔ **Give directions aloud.** You may want to make sure that you're alone — or else pretend that you're speaking to a cell phone. Repeat the information you want to remember out loud several times.

✔ **Keep important items somewhere visible.** Make sure that you place your medication and vitamins someplace where you can see them. If you have items that you want to take with you when you go out, put them in your car, in your bag, or by the door.

✔ **Keep everything well organized.** Go through files, drawers, and closets. Do you have so much clutter that you don't know where to begin? Hire a professional organizer. If money is an issue, get a friend or family member to help you.

> ✔ **Keep chores and errands to an absolute minimum.** Conserve your energy for the essentials: making sure that you're getting enough nutrients, eating small meals, and exercising.

Changing Successfully

Can you spare me some change, brother? No, not that kind of change. We're talking about modifying your behavior to attain a goal that's important to you. The problem? It's easier to stay with the status quo than to change a long-standing habit or try something new. Fortunately, after studying human behavior, psychologists have outlined a course of action that helps most anyone change successfully.

What follows is a simplified version of steps you can take to make it easier for you to revise your diet and lifestyle.

> ✔ **Take baby steps.** Break down the *target behavior* (the new behavior that you want to develop) into smaller, self-contained units. For example, you can write down each step that's entailed in changing your diet to a healthy one. It may be to start keeping a food journal, shopping for the right foods, cooking more at home, and so on. Approach each step as a separate mission (smaller goals that work toward the ultimate goal) and reward yourself whenever you accomplish them.
>
> ✔ **Identify elements in your environment that interfere with your target behavior.** After identifying what helps and what hinders, keep or increase what helps, and eliminate anything that hinders.
>
> ✔ **Eliminate the wrong foods.** This step is crucial in getting over hypoglycemia. Some people may be able to go cold turkey by giving up all their favorite foods and overhauling their lives overnight. For most people, it's much easier to change in degrees. See Chapter 6 for more info on maintaining a good diet.
>
> ✔ **Write down the consequences of continuing your current behavior.** Then write down all the benefits of reaching your goal. When you have a concrete picture of the positive results the new behavior can bring, you'll be more motivated to change to a healthier lifestyle.

Chapter 17

Ten-Plus Helpful Resources

This chapter shows you some of the more helpful hypoglycemia-related resources. These resources can help you find answers to many of the questions you may have.

The sources listed in this chapter aren't intended as an endorsement. The Internet isn't regulated, so use discretion and check more than one source for information. Remember that the Internet is constantly growing, so addresses and other information may change.

HELP: Institute for Body Chemistry

HELP, the Institute for Body Chemistry, was founded in 1979. This national network provides support and information for persons interested in body chemistry, especially as it relates to hypo-glycemia. It also promotes research between food and body chemistry, and provides assistance in starting support groups.

HELP, the Institute for Body Chemistry, P.O. Box 1338, Bryn Mawr, PA 19010; phone 610-525-1225.

The Hypoglycemia Association

The Hypoglycemia Association, Inc. (HAI) was founded in 1967. This international network provides literature, programs, bulletins, and meetings for people interested in hypoglycemia.

> Hypoglycemia Association, Inc., P.O. Box 165, Ashton, MD 20861-0165; phone 202-544-4044; Web site www.health.gov/NHIC/NHICScripts/Entry.cfm?HRCode=HR2253.

The Hypoglycemia Support Foundation, Inc.

The Hypoglycemia Support Foundation Web site provides products, diet information, surveys, and an on-line newsletter.

> The Hypoglycemia Support Foundation, Inc., P.O. Box 451778, Sunrise, FL 33345; Web site www.hypoglycemia.org.

Reactive Hypoglycemia Home Page

The Reactive Hypoglycemia Home Page gives you information about treatments that can help relieve the symptoms of hypoglycemia. It also provides a good list of resources for those wanting to find out more about the condition.

> Web site: www.fred.net/slowup/hypo.html.

Hypoglycemia Forum

The Hypoglycemia Forum Web site offers support and information to hypoglycemics and their family members. The site features a message board and several links to other helpful Web sites.

> Web site: http://hypoglycemia.itgo.com.

Hypoglycemia Homepage Holland

The Hypoglycemia Homepage Holland Web site offers general information about hypoglycemia, as well as health tips, a newsgroup, and lists of other helpful resources.

Web site: `http://hypoglykemie.nl`.

Ask the Dietitian

The hypoglycemia section of the Ask the Dietitian Web site features answers (from a registered and licensed dietitian) to a wide variety of questions about hypoglycemia-related topics.

Web site: `www.dietitian.com/hypoglyc.html`.

American Dietetic Association

You don't have to be a member to benefit from this site. Offers numerous healthy living tips, daily tips for healthy eating, nutrition fact sheets, weight management, vegetarian eating, answers to frequently asked questions about living a healthy lifestyle, and more.

American Dietetic Association, 216 W. Jackson Blvd. Chicago, IL 60606-6995; 312-899-0040; Web site: `www.eatright.org`

National Hypoglycemia Association

This nonprofit organization distributes literature and provides support for hypoglycemics and their families. It also provides medical, psychological, and nutritional referrals.

The National Hypoglycemia Association, P.O. Box 120, Ridgewood, NJ 07451; phone 201-670-1189.

Group Latino de Hipoglucemia

Group Latino de Hipoglucemia, Apdo. Postal 86-203, C.P. 14392, Mexico D.F.; phone 525 695-20-70

The Anxiety & Hypoglycemia Study Group

This group was founded by Professor J. H. Levitt in 1994. The group's purpose is to help educate people about the most common causes of biochemical imbalance.

Prof. J.H. Levitt of Pratt Institute (Brooklyn, NY); phone 212-479-7805; e-mail jlevitt@pratt.edu, Web site www.travelersonline.com/anxiety/.

Delphi Forums: Hypoglycemia Forum

This discussion board provides support and information to hypo-glycemics and their loved ones.

Web site: http://forums.delphiforums.com/hypoforum.

http://hypoglycemia.wordplay.org/

This Web site provides information on hypoglycemia, personal accounts from individuals who suffer from the condition, a discussion board, and links to other useful Web sites.

Depression Web Community

The Depression Web Community Web site offers information, help, and support for people who are depressed. The site features message boards, a chat room, and information about depression.

Web site: http://groups.msn.com/ DepressionWebCommunity.

Pain Net

The Pain Net Web site provides information about pain management, sources for information about pain and its causes, Pain Net News newsletters, listings for pain medicine practitioners in each state, a link to online counseling, and a bookstore.

Pain Net, Inc.; phone 614-481-5960, fax 614-481-5964; e-mail info@painnet.com, Web site www.painnet.com.

Vipassana Meditation Web Site

The Vipassana Meditation Web site offers information about Vipassana Meditation, worldwide course schedules, and a worldwide list of contacts.

Web site: www.dhamma.org.

Association for Traditional Studies

The Association for Traditional Studies Web site provides information about traditional studies, articles from the *Traditional Studies Journal,* a message board, and an online store. The site also offers information on the healing chi kung (Qigong) methods of Yin Style Ba Gua.

Association for Traditional Studies, 1630-A, 30th St., #420, Boulder, CO 80301; phone 303-440-5250, fax 303-440-5430; e-mail ats@traditionalstudies.org, Web site www.traditionalstudies.org.

Shake Off the Sugar

The Shake Off the Sugar Web site provides information, recipes, and products for cooking without sugar. It also features tools for determining the nutritional, protein, and sugar content of common foods.

Web site: www.shakeoffthesugar.net.

Glycemic Index (The Diabetes Mall)

The glycemic index section of The Diabetes Mall Web site helps you find the glycemic index of foods. The glycemic index measures how quickly a particular food is likely raise your blood sugar.

Web site: www.diabetesnet.com/diabetes_food_diet/glycemic_index.php.

Vegetarian Lowcarb (Immune Web)

The Vegetarian Lowcarb section of Immune Web shows vegetarians how to follow a low carbohydrate diet. It provides information on low-carb vegetable protein sources, products, menus, recipes, a mailing list, and links to other good resources.

Web site: http://immuneweb.org/lowcarb/.

The American Association of Naturopathic Physicians

The American Association of Naturopathic Physicians can help you find a naturopathic doctor near you. Naturopathic physicians treat hypoglycemia by finding the underlying cause for the condition rather than by just focusing on your symptoms. The Web site offers resources and information about naturopathic medicine.

The American Association of Naturopathic Physicians, 3201 New Mexico Ave., NW Suite 350, Washington, DC 20016; phone 866-538-2267 (toll free) or 202-895-1392, fax 202-274-1992; Web site www.naturopathic.org.

American Association for Health Freedom

The American Association for Health Freedom provides a political voice for health care providers who use a comprehensive approach, including nutritional therapies, preventative medical techniques, and natural treatments, when treating patients.

American Association for Health Freedom, 9912 Georgetown Pike, Suite D-2, P.O. Box 458, Great Falls, VA 32066; phone 800- 230-2762 or 703-759-0662, fax 703-759-6711; e-mail info@healthfreedom.net, Web site www.apma.net.

American Holistic Health Association (AHHA)

The American Holistic Health Association promotes the benefits of holistic principles. The AHHA Web site offers helpful resources, referral lists, self-help articles, and information about membership options.

The American Holistic Health Association, P.O. Box 17400, Anaheim, CA 92817-7400; phone 714-779-6152; e-mail mail@ahha.org, Web site www.ahha.org.

American Holistic Medical Association (AHMA)

The American Holistic Medical Association supports the professional and personal development of doctors as healers and educates them about the practice of holistic medicine. The AHMA Web site provides resources, links to other helpful Web sites, physician referrals, and membership information for doctors.

American Holistic Medical Association, 12101 Menaul Blvd. NE, Suite C, Albuquerque, NM 87112; phone 505-292-7788, fax 505-293-7582; e-mail info@holisticmedicine.org, Web site www.holisticmedicine.org.

The American College for Advancement in Medicine

The American College for Advancement in Medicine is dedicated to educating physicians in the latest advancements of preventative/nutritional medicine. The not-for-profit medical society's Web site features a book catalog, a database you can use to search for doctors, and membership information for doctors.

The American College for Advancement in Medicine, 23121 Verdugo Dr., Suite 204, Laguna Hills, CA 92653; fax 949-455-9679; Web site www.acam.org.

American Medical Association

The American Medical Association Web site offers doctor referrals, articles, and e-mail newsletters.

The American Medical Association, 515 N. State St., Chicago, IL 60610; phone 312-464-5000; Web site www.ama-assn.org.

American Medical Women's Association

The American Medical Woman's Association Web site features health topics of concern to women, a list of helpful publications, links to other informative Web sites, a bookstore, and membership information for doctors and students.

The American Medical Women's Association, 801 N. Fairfax St., Suite 400, Alexandria, VA 22314; phone 703-838-0500, fax 703-549-3864; e-mail info@amwa-doc.org, Web site www. amwa doc.org.

American Dietetic Association

The American Dietetic Association Web site provides a nationwide dietitian referral service, information and tips for maintaining good nutrition, listings of good resources, a catalog of products and services, and membership information for doctors and students.

American Dietetic Association, 216 W. Jackson Blvd., Chicago, IL 60606-6995; phone 312-899-0040; Web site www. eatright.org.

Seeds of Change

The Seeds of Change Web site offers organic garden seeds and natural products, organic gardening advice, e-mail newsletters, and a garden help forum.

Seeds of Change, P.O. Box 15700, Santa Fe, NM 87506; phone 888-762-7333; e-mail gardener@seedsofchange.com, Web site http://store.yahoo.com/seedsofchange.

Body Ecology

The Body Ecology Web site is a good source for stevia and books with sugar-free recipes that use the sweetener.

Body Ecology, 273 Fairway Dr., Asheville, NC 28805; phone 800-511-2660 (U.S.) or 800-896-7838 (Canada), fax 770-234-5453; Web site www.bodyecology.net.

nSpired Natural Foods

The nSpired Natural Foods Web site offers a variety of natural (and/or organic) foods, including Pumpkorn, an all-natural snack food made from pumpkin seeds.

nSpired Natural Foods, 14855 Wicks Blvd., San Leandro, CA 94577; phone 510-686-0116, fax 510-686-0126; e-mail info@nspiredfoods.com, Web site www.nspiredfoods.com.

Herbal Advantage, Inc.

Herbal Advantage, Inc. sells stevia and other herbs, spices, and natural items.

Herbal Advantage, Inc., 131 Bobwhite Rd., Rogersville, MO 65742; phone 800-753-9199 or 417-753-4000, fax 417-753-2000; e-mail info@herbaladvantage.com, Web site www.herbaladvantage.com.

Northwest Natural

Northwest Natural markets frozen fish products that are convenient sources of beneficial Omega-3 fatty acids. The company makes salmon burgers, halibut burgers, and tuna with pesto medallions.

Phone: 360-866-9661.

Bob's Red Mill Natural Foods

Bob's Red Mill sells natural stone ground whole grains, such as flours, cereals, meals, bulk grains, seeds, and beans.

Bob's Red Mill Natural Foods, 5209 NE International Way, Milwaukie, OR 97222; phone 800-349-2173, fax 503-653-1339;Web site www.bobsredmill.com.

Metagenics

The Metagenics Web site offers vitamins and supplements, as well as information on nutrition.

Metagenics, Inc., 166 Fernwood Ave., Adison, NH 08837; phone 800-692-9400; Web site www.metagenics.com.

Thorne Research, Inc.

The Thorne Research Web site offers high-quality nutritional supplements, an alternative medicine review, and a quarterly newsletter.

Thorne Research, Inc., P.O. Box 25, Dover, ID 83825; phone 208-263-1337, fax 208-265-2488; Web site www.thorne.com.

www.syndrome-x.com

This Web site provides information on Syndrome X, a group of health problems that can include insulin resistance, abnormal blood fats, overweight, and high blood pressure.

USDA Food and Nutrition Information Center

The USDA Food and Nutrition Information Center Web site provides information about food, nutrition, and food safety. The site offers a large variety of resources, links, and databases that deal with the topics of food and nutrition.

Food and Nutrition Information Center, Agricultural Research Service, USDA National Agricultural Library, Room 105, 10301 Baltimore Ave., Beltsville, MD 20705-2351; phone 301-504-5719, TTY 301-504-6856, fax 301-504-6409; e-mail fnic@nal.usda.gov, Web site www.nal.usda.gov/fnic.

Herb Research Foundation

The Herb Research Foundation provides science-based information on the safety and benefits of herbs, as well as information on the sustainable development of botanical resources. The foundation's Web site offers a wide variety of resources, links, and information on herbs.

Herb Research Foundation, 1007 Pearl St., Suite 200, Boulder, CO 80302; phone 303-449-2265 (office) or 800-748-2617 (voice mail), fax 303-449-7849; e-mail info@herbs.org, Web site www.herbs.org.

American Botanical Council

The American Botanical Council provides science-based information that promotes the safe use of herbal medicines. The council's Web site has information on herbs, a list of resources, and critical reviews of current journal articles.

American Botanical Council, 6200 Manor Rd., Austin, TX 78714-4345; phone 512-926-4900, fax 512-926-2345; e-mail abc@herbalgram.org, Web site www.herbalgram.org.

MayoClinic.com

The MayoClinic.com Web site offers useful information and interactive tools to help you better understand and manage your health.

The site also features answers from readers' questions and a newsletter.

Web site: www.mayoclinic.com.

American Diabetes Association

The American Diabetes Association Web site provides information on diabetes, guidelines for healthy living, recipes, an E-newsletter, and an online store.

The American Diabetes Association, 1701 North Beauregard St., Alexandria, VA 22311; phone 800-342-2383; Web site www.diabetes.org.

CDC Diabetes Public Health Resource

The CDC Diabetes Public Health Resource Web site provides a wide assortment of information and resources on diabetes. The Web site also has links to other good sources of information.

CDC Division of Diabetes Translation, P.O. Box 8728, Silver Spring, MD 20910; phone 877-232-3422, fax 301-562-1050; e-mail diabetes@cdc.gov, Web site www.cdc.gov/diabetes.

American Obesity Association

The American Obesity Association focuses its efforts on changing public policies and perceptions about obesity. The association's Web site offers information about obesity, consumer protection, prevention of weight gain, treatments for obesity, and discrimination. It also talks about current research on the subject of obesity.

American Obesity Association, 1250 24th St., NW, Suite 300, Washington, DC 20037; phone 202-776-7711, fax 202-776-7712; Web site www.obesity.org.

National Qigong Association

The National Qigong Association Web site features member listings, a discussion board, information, a newsletter, links, and a guide to current events the NQA is involved in.

> National Qigong Association, P.O. Box 540, Ely, MN 55731; phone 218-365-6330, fax 218-365-6933; e-mail info@nqa.org, Web site www.nqa.org.

Organic Consumers Association

The Organic Consumers Association campaigns for food safety, organic agriculture, fair trade, and sustainability. The association's Web site provides information about organic foods and food safety, listings for food safety events and conferences, a Greenpeople directory for listings of organic food producers and suppliers, and newsletters, fact sheets, and campaign materials.

> Organic Consumers Association, 6101 Cliff Estate Rd., Little Marais, MN 55614; phone 218-226-4164, fax 218-226-4157; Web site http://organicconsumers.org.

Vegetarian Resource Group (VRG)

The Vegetarian Resource Group is a non-profit organization that focuses on educating the public about vegetarianism and related issues, such as health, nutrition, ecology, ethics, and world hunger. The VRG Web site offers information on vegetarianism and veganism, recipes, a newsletter, links to other good Web sites, a bulletin board, excerpts from the *Vegetarian Journal,* and an online book catalog.

> The Vegetarian Resource Group (VRG), P.O. Box 1463, Dept. IN, Baltimore, MD 21203; phone 410-366-8343; e-mail vrg@vrg.org, Web site www.vrg.org.

Health Equations

Health Equations provides nutritional blood testing. The Health Equations Web site offers information about the testing, as well as articles on topics such as cholesterol and heart disease.

Health Equations, P.O. Box 323, Newfane, VT 05345; phone 802-365-9213, fax 802-365-9218; Web site www. healthequations.com.

Great Smokies Diagnostic Laboratories

The Great Smokies Diagnostic Laboratories can perform food-allergy tests. The Great Smokies Diagnostic Laboratories Web site offers information about the different tests the laboratory performs, news about latest lab developments, educational resources, an online bookstore, and a newsletter.

Great Smokies Diagnostic Laboratories, 63 Zillicoa St., Asheville, NC 28801; phone 800-522-4762, fax 828-252-9303; Web site www.gsdl.com.

Community Support Group for Hypoglycemics

To get a self-help support group started in your community or to locate one already established, send a self-addressed, stamped envelope and your name, street address, and phone number to

Franklin Publishers, Box 1338, Bryn Mawr, PA 19010

Index

• C •

caffeine
 alternatives for, 182–183, 232
 avoiding, 80, 232
 effects of, 23, 195
calcium
 absorption of, with spinach, 82
 dosage of, 101, 102
 for insomnia, 113
 for stress, 116
California poppy, 117
candidiasis, 31–32
carbohydrate density (CD), 88
carbohydrate intolerance, 9
carbohydrates
 addiction to, 23
 affect on blood sugar level, 18–19, 74
 breads and grains, 86–90
 complex, 17, 87
 cravings for, 23, 74, 75, 137
 definition, 17
 digestion of, 21
 exercise requirements for, 122–123
 fruit, 80–81
 GI (glycemic index) for, 88–89
 legumes, 87
 percentage in hypoglycemic diet,
  77, 93
 produced during digestion, 16
 simple (refined), 11, 17, 87
 symptoms of eating too little, 77–78
 vegetables, 81–84
carbonated beverages, avoiding, 80
carob, 182–183
Cash, Adam (*Psychology For
  Dummies*), 149
cayenne pepper, 116
CD (carbohydrate density), 88
CDC Diabetes Public Health
  Resource, 246
CFS. *See* chronic fatigue syndrome
chamomile, 117
change, dealing with, 234
chasteberry, 114
chatterbox, 27
check-ups. *See* physical exams

cheese. *See also* dairy foods
 processed, avoiding, 80
 serving size for, 92
chewing gum, 231
chicken, recipe for, 220–221
children. *See* family
Chinese medicine. *See* TCM
chocolate
 carob as substitute for, 182–183
 phenylethylamine in, 148
cholesterol
 avocados reducing, 83
 garlic and onions reducing, 83
 ginger reducing, 115
 insulin resistance and, 34
 Syndrome X and, 35
choline, 114
chromium, 101, 116
chronic fatigue syndrome (CFS), 32,
  105–106, 110–111. *See also*
  fatigue
chutney, recipe for, 214–215
cigarettes. *See* nicotine
cinnamon, 116
circular thinking, 29
circulation, poor, 33, 116. *See also*
  cold hands and feet
CLA (Conjugated linolenic acid),
  103
Clinistix, 226
coffee. *See* caffeine
cognitive coping skills, 151
cognitive patterns, changing, 150
cold hands and feet, 27. *See also*
  circulation, poor
Cold Poached Salmon with Fresh
  Fruit Chutney and Herb Sauce
  recipe, 214–215
Community Support Group for
  Hypoglycemics, 248
complex carbohydrates, 17, 87
comprehensive treatment, 127
concentration, problems with, 29, 30,
  32, 114
conditions related to hypoglycemia.
  See related conditions to
  hypoglycemia

restlessness, 29
riboflavin, 101
rice pilaf, recipe for, 207
ringing in ears, 27
Rinzler, Carol Ann (*Controlling Cholesterol For Dummies*), 83
Roast Chicken with Red Onions and Potatoes recipe, 220–221
Roasted Red Pepper Dip recipe, 206–207
Roasted Vegetable Salsa recipe, 218–219
rosemary tea, 114
Rubin, Alan L., MD
　Diabetes Cookbook For Dummies, 12, 93
　Diabetes For Dummies, 36
running as exercise, 125–126

• S •

salad, oriental, recipe for, 209
saliva, role in digestion, 16
salmon, recipe for, 214–215
salsa, recipes for, 212–213, 218–219
salted green soybeans, 230
SAM-e (S-adenosyl-methionine), 106, 108, 112
saturated fats, 84
saw palmetto, 114
Schlosberg, Susanne (*Fitness For Dummies*), 122
sea vegetables, 83–84
seaweed (nori), 230
Seeds of Change, 243
selenium, 102, 107, 116
self-awareness, 159–161
self-hypnosis, 142–144
serotonin, 148, 152–153, 230
serving sizes, 91–92
sex drive, low, 29, 113–114
Shake Off the Sugar web site, 239
shakiness, 1, 9
shrimp, recipe for, 216–217
Siberian ginseng, 105, 111
simple (refined) carbohydrates, 11, 17, 87
skullcap, 104

sleep disorders, 31, 34. *See also* insomnia
smoking. *See* nicotine
snacks
　before bed, 36
　content of, 196
　before dining out, 227
　before exercise, 125
　GI (glycemic index) for, 89
　keeping with you, 182, 225
　number of per day, 12, 90
　protein included in, 75
　scheduling based on lab test results, 45
　vegetables and nuts as, 230–231
soft drinks, avoiding, 80
sore throat, 32
soup, recipe for, 208, 212–213
soy foods, 93–94
soybeans, salted green, 230
specialists, 61–63
Spinach Pie recipe, 210
spouse. *See* family
sprouts, 83
SSRI (Selective Serotonin Reuptake Inhibitors), 152
St. John's Wort, 108
starch, removing from foods, 229. *See also* carbohydrates
Staud, Roland, MD (*Fibromyalgia For Dummies*), 31, 111
stevia, 228, 230, 243
stinging nettle, 111, 115
stomach, digestive problems and, 109
stress
　breathing techniques for, 136–138
　Holmes-Rahe Social Adjustment Rating Scale for, 134
　low tolerance for, 29
　meditation for, 138–142
　relationship to hypoglycemia, 10, 139
　relaxation techniques for, 134–136
　self-hypnosis for, 142–144
　vitamins and supplements for, 116–117
　work-related, 180–184
string beans, 83

Notes

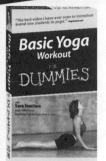
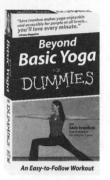
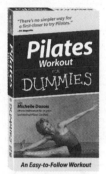
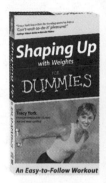
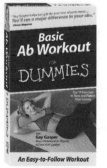
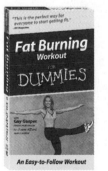
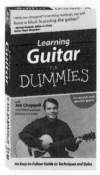

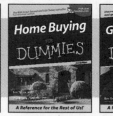

FOR DUMMIES®

Helping you expand your horizons and realize your potential

PERSONAL FINANCE & BUSINESS

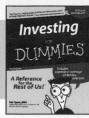

Investing
0-7645-2431-3

Home Buying
0-7645-5331-3

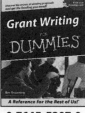

Grant Writing
0-7645-5307-0

Also available:

Accounting For Dummies
(0-7645-5314-3)

Business Plans Kit For Dummies
(0-7645-5365-8)

Managing For Dummies
(1-5688-4858-7)

Mutual Funds For Dummies
(0-7645-5329-1)

QuickBooks All-in-One Desk Reference For Dummies
(0-7645-1963-8)

Resumes For Dummies
(0-7645-5471-9)

Small Business Kit For Dummies
(0-7645-5093-4)

Starting an eBay Business For Dummies
(0-7645-1547-0)

Taxes For Dummies 2003
(0-7645-5475-1)

HOME, GARDEN, FOOD & WINE

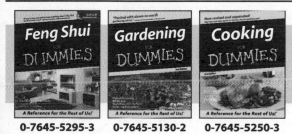

Feng Shui
0-7645-5295-3

Gardening
0-7645-5130-2

Cooking
0-7645-5250-3

Also available:

Bartending For Dummies
(0-7645-5051-9)

Christmas Cooking For Dummies
(0-7645-5407-7)

Cookies For Dummies
(0-7645-5390-9)

Diabetes Cookbook For Dummies
(0-7645-5230-9)

Grilling For Dummies
(0-7645-5076-4)

Home Maintenance For Dummies
(0-7645-5215-5)

Slow Cookers For Dummies
(0-7645-5240-6)

Wine For Dummies
(0-7645-5114-0)

FITNESS, SPORTS, HOBBIES & PETS

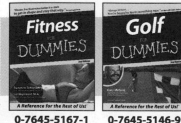

Fitness
0-7645-5167-1

Golf
0-7645-5146-9

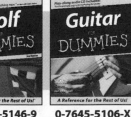

Guitar
0-7645-5106-X

Also available:

Cats For Dummies
(0-7645-5275-9)

Chess For Dummies
(0-7645-5003-9)

Dog Training For Dummies
(0-7645-5286-4)

Labrador Retrievers For Dummies
(0-7645-5281-3)

Martial Arts For Dummies
(0-7645-5358-5)

Piano For Dummies
(0-7645-5105-1)

Pilates For Dummies
(0-7645-5397-6)

Power Yoga For Dummies
(0-7645-5342-9)

Puppies For Dummies
(0-7645-5255-4)

Quilting For Dummies
(0-7645-5118-3)

Rock Guitar For Dummies
(0-7645-5356-9)

Weight Training For Dummies
(0-7645-5168-X)

Available wherever books are sold.
Go to www.dummies.com or call 1-877-762-2974 to order direct

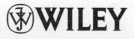

WILEY

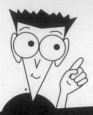

FOR DUMMIES®

A world of resources to help you grow

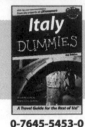
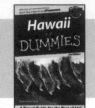
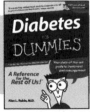
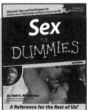
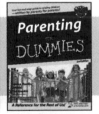